MW01122373

INTERPROFESSIONAL CLIENT-CENTRED COLLABORATIVE PRACTICE

WHAT DOES IT LOOK LIKE? HOW CAN IT BE ACHIEVED?

PROFESSIONS - TRAINING, EDUCATION AND DEMOGRAPHICS

Additional books in this series can be found on Nova's website under the Series tab.

Additional e-books in this series can be found on Nova's website under the e-book tab.

PROFESSIONS - TRAINING, EDUCATION AND DEMOGRAPHICS

INTERPROFESSIONAL CLIENT-CENTRED COLLABORATIVE PRACTICE

WHAT DOES IT LOOK LIKE?
HOW CAN IT BE ACHIEVED?

CAROLE ORCHARD & LESLEY BAINBRIDGE
CO-EDITORS

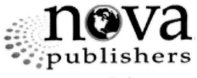

New York

Library of Congress Cataloging-in-Publication Data

Names: Orchard, Carole.
Title: Interprofessional client-centred collaborative practice : what does it
  look like? how can it be achieved? / editors: Carole Orchard (Associate
  Professor, Office of Interprofessional Health Education & Research, G22
  Siebens Drake Research Institute, Western University, London, Ontario,
  Canada).
Description: Hauppauge, New York : Nova Science Publisher's, Inc., 2015. |
  Series: Professions - training, education and demographics | Includes
  indexes.
Identifiers: LCCN 2015032796 | ISBN 9781634837545 (hardcover)
Subjects: LCSH: Medical personnel and patient. | Interpersonal communication.
Classification: LCC R727.3 .I59 2015 | DDC 610.69/6--dc23 LC record available at
http://lccn.loc.gov/2015032796

Published by Nova Science Publishers, Inc. † *New York*

CONTENTS

Foreword   vii

Acknowledgments   ix

Author Biographies   xi

Introduction to Interprofessional Client-Centered Collaborative Practice –
A Practical Primer for Educators in the Practice Setting   xvii

Chapter 1   Towards a Framework of Client-Centered Collaborative Practice   1
Carole Orchard

Chapter 2   What Is Competence in Client-Centered Collaborative Practice?   17
Carole Orchard and Lesley Bainbridge

Chapter 3   Perioperative Practice in the Context of Client-Centered Care   37
Marion Jones, Isabel Jamieson and Leigh Anderson

Chapter 4   Should There Be an *"I"* in Team?
A New Perspective on Developing and Maintaining
Collaborative Networks in Health Professional Care   51
Lesley Bainbridge and Glenn Regehr

Chapter 5   Changing Organizational Culture to Embrace
Interprofessional Education and Interprofessional Practice   67
Ivy Oandasan

Chapter 6   Engaging Health Professionals in Continuing
Interprofessional Development   83
Jill Thistlethwaite

Chapter 7   The Effect of Leadership Support on Interprofessional Practice,
Team Effectiveness, and Patient Safety Outcomes   95
*Heather K. S. Laschinger, Brenda J. Stutsky
and Emily A. Read*

Chapter 8   Transformative Interprofessional Continuing Education
and Professional Development to Meet Client Care Needs:
A Synthesis of Best Practices   113
*Rosemary Brander, Lesley Bainbridge,
Janice P. Van Dijk and Margo Paterson*

Chapter 9   Theory into Practice: The Challenges and Rewards
                    of Developing and Running an Interprofessional Health Clinic   **131**
                    Daniel O'Brien and Marion Jones

Chapter 10   Moving from Atheoretical to Theoretical Approaches
                    to Interprofessional Client-Centered Collaborative Practice   **143**
                    Sarah Hean, Shelley Doucet, Lesley Bainbridge,
                    Valerie Ball, Liz Anderson, Clive Baldwin, Chris Green,
                    Richard Pitt, Stefanus Snyman, Mattie Schmidtt,
                    Phil Clark, John Gilbert and Ivy Oandasan

Chapter 11   Evaluation of Continuing Interprofessional Client-Centered
                    Collaborative Practice Programs   **161**
                    Carole Orchard

Chapter 12   Assessment of Learning within Interprofessional Client-Centered
                    Collaborative Practice –Challenges and Solutions   **171**
                    Carole Orchard

Author Index   **189**

Subject Index   **197**

FOREWORD

Interprofessional client-centered collaborative practice (ICCCP) is collective by nature, emerging as it does at the intersection of a wide variety of professional knowledge and scopes of practice. Many studies of ICCCP focus on the determinants or inputs of collaborative practice as well as on the results, outputs, or outcomes. This is echoed methodologically, as a preponderance of ICCCP teamwork studies primarily employ interview and survey data. However, close observations are also necessary to build understanding of the collective behavioral processes of interprofessional collaboration. Many authors point out the need for more studies of the actual *practices* of collaboration. In many senses, ICCCP represents what Rittel and Webber (1973) have called a "wicked" problem. (p. 155) Wicked problems are "difficult or impossible to solve. Their solutions depend on incomplete, contradictory and changing requirements that are often difficult to recognize. And they are confounded by complex interdependencies between actors and agents." (Drinka & Clark, 2000, p. 37) If ever there was a wicked problem, innovation in ICCCP is surely one. As a series of possible solutions to this problem, the various case studies set out in this monograph are welcomed.

Learning to become a competent health professional has always been a two-part process – that which focuses on 'classroom' teaching and that which engages students in an apprenticeship with qualified professionals in real-world settings. Universities, colleges, and institutes depend upon practice settings for the apprenticeship education of their health professional students. Practice education (PE) settings require competent health care professionals to deliver quality care to patients. Until recently, the delivery of health profession education has been almost entirely discipline based, with each discipline educating their own students in isolation – whether on campus or in the community. As is clear in this book, there is now increasing emphasis on all health care professions to learn how to be competent collaborators. This emerging shift in education has led to a new interest in different approaches to the delivery of health professional education, approaches that embrace more opportunities for interactions amongst and between learners across health and human service/social care professions. PE settings are being recognized as ideal environments for interprofessional education (IPE), in which students can witness and practice how to work interprofessionally with others on healthcare teams — that is, to learn about, with, and from each other, for the purpose of collaboration to improve quality of care. The chapters in this book focus on the many issues that confront healthcare professionals in their efforts to provide true interprofessional collaborative care, with the patient or client as the center of focus.

The term *practice* tends to occupy a black box in interprofessional literature. Although it is frequently invoked in considerations of collaboration, teamwork, and team working, it is seldom explicitly defined. One exception comes from Thistlethwaite, Jackson, and Moran (2013), who suggested that practice can be understood in three ways: (a) as the enactment of a role or profession, (b) as a moment of collective unity or performance, and/or (c) as a "socially institutionalized and socially acceptable form of interaction requiring cognitive understanding and reflection." (p. 54) This book deals in a number of ways with these three ideas, thus providing a better understanding of the term *practice* by removing it from a black box and placing it within our concept of a partnership between a team of healthcare providers.

It is now recognized that effective ICCCP requires the active engagement of students from different professions using interactive learning methodologies to develop health professional students' knowledge, skills, attitudes, perceptions, and behaviors. As noted in this book, ICCCP requires a complex adult learning (andragogy) approach that is most effective when integrated throughout a program of study, moving from simple to more complex learning activities that bridge from post-secondary to practice education settings. Educational accreditation standards being developed to stimulate the advancement of IPE will have an impact on policies in both the academic and clinical settings that encompass ICCCP.

Continuing professional development (CPD) is an integral part of the learning continuum to ensure that ICCCP is built on a theory-informed base and sustained in changing healthcare environments. This book will serve as a much-needed primer to inform CPD in all aspects of ICCCP. The thoughtful and clearly articulated chapters contained here are, therefore, most welcome practical guides for practice educators, and a very useful source of information for a broader audience of healthcare providers who are faced with the complex issues that confront enactment of true ICCCP.

John H. V. Gilbert, C.M., Ph.D., FCAHS
Vancouver
2015

REFERENCES

Drinka, T.J.K., & Clark, P.G., (2000). Health care teamwork: Interdisciplinary practice and teaching. Westport, Conneticut: Auburn House.

Rittel, H. W. J., & Webber, M. M. (1973). Dilemmas in a general theory of planning. *Policy Sciences, 4*, 155–169. http://dx.doi.org/10.1007/BF01405730

Thistlethwaite, J., Jackson, A., & Moran, M. (2013). Interprofessional collaborative practice: A deconstruction. *Journal of Interprofessional Care, 27*, 50–56. http://dx.doi.org/10.3109/13561820.2012.730075

ACKNOWLEDGMENTS

This book would not have been possible without the significant contributions in our understanding that have occurred over the past decade or so. Insights provided from many clients and their families, learners in both pre- and post-licensure programs, and colleagues have assisted in helping the authors of this book's chapters in how we can move towards a more all-inclusive approach to improve the care and services delivered to others. We also wish to acknowledge many in our respective communities who have challenged our thinking through their thought-provoking questions. Hence this book is truly a collaborative effort from many. We are the privileged who are allowed to share our synthesis of all this learning.

We also would be remiss without thanking our colleagues who so willingly agreed to share their insights and learning, and findings form their own experiential and research work. Furthermore, this book could not be completed without the wisdom and skills of Shanaya McKay of Amay Editing Inc. We both learned a great deal of the in-depth application of APA and improving the way we express thoughts from her.

And to our colleagues at NOVA Publishing who have guided us through the process of moving a set of chapters around a key topic of interest to the field of interprofessional education and collaborative practice into a publishable book. Thank you to everyone!

Carole Orchard
Lesley Bainbridge

AUTHOR BIOGRAPHIES

Orchard, Carole A., BSN, MEd., EdD.

Dr. Orchard is currently Professor and Coordinator of Interprofessional Health Education & Research for the Faculty of Health Sciences and the Schulich School of Medicine & Dentistry at the University of Western Ontario. Her research focuses on interprofessional patient centred collaborative practice. Dr. Orchard and her colleagues have developed two measurement instruments: Interprofessional Socialization & Valuing Scale (ISVS) and the Assessment of Interprofessional Team Collaboration Scale (AITCS). Dr. Orchard was also a member of the Canadian Interprofessional Health Collaborative Steering Committee (CIHC) until 2010 and co-chaired its IP Competency Working Group who developed the CIHC National IP Competency Framework.

Bainbridge, Lesley A., BSR(PT), MEd, PhD

Dr. Bainbridge holds a master's degree in education and an interdisciplinary doctoral degree with a focus on interprofessional health education. She served as Associate Principal, College of Health Disciplines and Director, Interprofessional Education, Faculty of Medicine at the University of British Columbia from 2005 to 2015 and 2014 respectively. She was also an Associate Professor, Department of Physical Therapy at UBC. Dr. Bainbridge has been principal or co-investigator on several Teaching and Learning Enhancement Fund grants, two major Health Canada grants focusing on interprofessional education and collaborative practice and other funded research related to interprofessional education and collaborative practice. She has published in peer reviewed journals and presented on IPE related topics at national and international conferences. She retired from the University on June 30, 2015 and remains involved with graduate students, short term projects and interprofessional developments locally, nationally and internationally.

Jones, Marion, PhD, RGON, M.Ed. (Admin) (Hons), BA, M.Ed. (Admin) (Hons)

Professor Marion Jones is Dean of University Postgraduate Studies at Auckland University of Technology, a director of the National Centre for Interprofessional Education and Collaborative Practice in New Zealand and Professor of Interprofessional Education at the University of Derby in the United Kingdom. A significant focus of her academic career has been the development of post graduate study. For ten years she provided her expertise as Associate Dean Postgraduate to the Faculty of Health and Environmental Sciences. Her area of research expertise and publication is interprofessional practice and education, postgraduate supervision and perioperative nursing. Her latest publications include co editing three books on Interprofessional leadership. Her PhD examined the shaping of interprofessional practice in the context of health reform. Some of her national and international activities include being a board member of InterEd, the New Zealand representative on the Australasian Interprofessional Practice & Education Network (AIPPEN), fellow of the College of Nurses Aotearoa CAN (NZ) and auditor for The Academic Quality Agency for New Zealand Universities (AQA).

Oandasan, Ivy, MD, MHSc, CCFP, FCFP

Ivy Oandasan is Full Professor with the Department of Family and Community Medicine at the University of Toronto. An active family physician who practices at the Toronto Western Hospital she has been involved in teaching and research since 1997. Passionate about enhancing the education provided to health professional learners, Dr. Oandasan's main scholarly area has been in curriculum development and research related to community oriented primary care, health advocacy and interprofessional education. In January of 2006, Dr. Oandasan was named the inaugural Director of the Office of Interprofessional Education at the University of Toronto (U of T). In this role she was able to catalyze relationships within and across hospitals and the university health science faculties to advance interprofessional education (IPE) and interprofessional care (IPC). She was Co-Chair for HealthForceOntario's Interprofessional Blueprint for Action that advanced a systems approach to implement IPE and IPC across Ontario and led the national research team funded by Health Canada that developed a theoretical framework used worldwide on Interprofessionality: the field of study exploring interprofessional practice and interprofessional education. In her most recent position as The Director of Education at the College of Family Physicians of Canada (CFPC), the national certifying and accrediting body for family medicine, she is charged with enhancing undergraduate and postgraduate family medicine education supporting the development of family physicians who can meet societal needs. Dr. Oandasan's burning educational platform remains to foster a generation of competent and caring healthcare professionals who believe in the practice of interprofessional patient-centered care. She grounds her knowledge and practice through her work as a clinician, educator, researcher, administrator, and leader.

Regehr, Glenn, PhD

Glenn Regehr obtained his PhD in cognitive science from McMaster University then spent one year as a Research Associate in medical education at the McMaster University Program for Education Research and Development. In 1993 he joined the University of Toronto, Faculty of Medicine as Assistant Professor.

During his career as a researcher in the field of health professions education, Dr. Regehr has been involved in founding of, and held leadership positions at, The University of Toronto Wilson Centre for Research in Education, The University of Ottawa Academy for Innovation in Medical Education and the University of British Columbia Centre for Health Education Scholarship. Since 2009 he has been Associate Director (Research) for CHES and Professor at UBC.

Through his various research collaborations, he has co-authored over 200 peer reviewed papers on topics including: OSCE measures, authentic clinical assessment, professionalism, professional identity formation, self-assessment and feedback. In addition to over 20 awards for individual papers and presentations, his career awards include the NBME Hubbard Award (2007), the MCC Award for Outstanding Achievement in the Evaluation of Clinical Competence (2008), the CAME Ian Hart Award for Distinguished Contribution to Medical Education (2013) and the CAME Early Career Medical Educators Mentorship Award (2015).

Thistlethwaite, Jill, BSc, MBBS, PhD, MMEd, FRCGP, FRACGP

Professor Jill Thistlethwaite is a health professions education consultant and general practitioner, adjunct professor at University of Technology Sydney and academic title holder at the University of Queensland. She trained as a GP in the UK and has worked as a health professional academic in the UK and Australia. Her research interests include interprofessional education and practice, professionalism, shared decision making and women's health. She has published extensively in health education and clinical practice, has written or co-authored five books, co-edited four, several book chapters and about 100 peer-reviewed papers. She is co-editor in chief of The Clinical Teacher and an associate editor of the Journal of Interprofessional Care. In 2014 Professor Thistlethwaite was a Fulbright senior scholar at the National Center for Interprofessional Practice and Education at the University of Minnesota, USA.

Hean, Sarah, PhD

Dr. Hean is an associate professor in the School of Health & Social Care at Bournemouth University in the U.K. and also the Marie Curie-Sklodowsk Fellow with the University of Stavanger in Norway. She brings a sociologist's perspective to IPC. She has served on the CAIPE Board and is the Associate Editor of the Journal of Interprofessional Care and chair of the In-2- Theory: Interprofessional Scholarship, Education and Practice on Facebook.

O'Brien, Daniel, BHSc. (Physiotherapy), PGDip, MHSc. (Hons.),

Daniel O'Brien is a lecturer in the physiotherapy department at Auckland University of Technology (AUT). He trained as physiotherapist at AUT and after spending six years working in private practice both in New Zealand and the UK, moved into clinical education and academia. He is currently undertaking his PhD., which is looking at patients' and clinicians' beliefs regarding the management of osteoarthritis. His other research interests include facilitating behaviour change in healthcare, and exploring interprofessional collaboration in healthcare practice.

Laschinger, Heather Spence K.

Dr. Laschinger is a Professor in the Arthur Labatt School of Nursing at the University of Western Ontario in London, Ontario, Canada. For the past 25 years, Dr. Laschinger has been investigating the impact of nursing work environments on nurses' empowerment for professional practice, their health and well-being, and the role of leadership in creating empowering working conditions. A major focus of Dr. Laschinger's research is examining the link between nursing work environments and nurse and client outcomes. The results of this research have been translated into several policy documents, including the Magnet Hospital Accreditation Program in the USA. Research findings have also been used to inform workplace practices in healthcare work settings worldwide. In 2009, Dr. Laschinger was awarded the Arthur Labatt Family Nursing Research Chair in Health Human Resources Optimization to lead a broad research agenda examining issues related to the planning and management of nursing and health services to ensure high quality care across healthcare sectors. She has received several prestigious national and international awards for her work in academic and professional communities, including the Distinguished University Professor Award and Hellmuth Prize at Western University and fellowships in the Canadian Academy of Health Sciences and the American Academy of Nursing. Dr. Laschinger has also been appointed by the Ontario Minister of Heather as Healthy Work Environment Champion for the province.

Stutsky, Brenda J. RN, BN, MScN, EdS, PhD

Dr. Stutsky is the Director of Organization and Staff Development with the Northern Health Region, Manitoba, Canada. She also works with the Manitoba Practice Assessment Program for physicians in the Faculty of Health Sciences, University of Manitoba, Canada. In addition, she holds appointments as an Assistant Professor with the Colleges of Nursing and Medicine in the Faculty of Health Sciences, University of Manitoba. In 2009, Dr. Stutsky completed her PhD in Computing Technology in Education from Nova Southeastern University, Fort Lauderdale, Florida, USA where she studied leadership development in an online learning community. In 2012, Dr. Stutsky completed a post-doctoral fellowship in Health Human Resource Optimization at the University of Western Ontario where she created and tested a conceptual framework for interprofessional collaborative practice. As a registered nurse of 32 years, she is keenly aware of the positive outcomes of interprofessional practice on patient care and safety and incorporates competencies of interprofessional practice into region-wide clinical and leadership education programs.

Brander, Rosemary Ph.D., M.Sc., B.Sc. (PT)

Dr. Brander is Director, Office of Interprofessional Education & Practice, and Assistant Professor, School of Rehabilitation Therapy at Queen's University, Kingston, Ontario, Canada. She is also the Senior Researcher & Program Evaluator, Centre for Studies in Aging & Health at Providence Care, Kingston. Her research interests include collaborative practice and customer service in healthcare environments, interprofessional education and collaborative leadership, and organizational change for improved health outcomes. She was the co-lead for Queen's University on the Canadian Interprofessional Health Leadership Collaborative from 2012-2015.

Dr. Brander holds a doctorate in Rehabilitation Sciences from Queen's University, a Master of Science from the University of Western Ontario, and a Bachelor of Science (Physical Therapy) from Queen's University. Her doctoral dissertation is entitled "Collaborative Care Relations: Examining Perspectives for Application and Change in a Canadian Hospital." She has held a variety of health leadership roles and has extensive experience as a clinical physiotherapist working with children and adults with long-term neurologic disabilities.

Anderson, Leigh, RN

Leigh Anderson is a Registered Nurse who is currently working in the role of Project Manager at Auckland District Health Board. Leigh has held various roles throughout her nursing career and was most recently Perioperative Nurse Consultant. In the last 3 years Leigh has diversified into performance improvement and completed her Green Belt (Lean 6 Sigma) training. Leigh has held professional positions with the Perioperative Nurses College of NZNO working regionally and internationally as Chairperson and also representing the College on the Board of the International Federation of Perioperative Nurses.

Jamieson, Isabel, RN, PhD, MNurse(Melb), CertAT,

Dr. Jamieson is currently employed by the Christchurch Polytechnic Institution of Technology (CPIT), Department of Nursing and Human Service (NHS) as a senior nursing lecturer and adjunct senior fellow, University of Canterbury, Christchurch New Zealand. Other roles include Chair of the NHS research committee, member of the CPIT ethics committee, thesis supervisor and thesis examiner. Her research interests include health care workforce issues, clinical models of teaching and learning, nursing student's readiness to practice as well as the graduate nurse experience.

Isabel's clinical background is perioperative nursing, surgical assisting and infection control. She is currently Chair of the Professional and Education Committee of the New Zealand Nurses Organization Perioperative Nurses College.

Paterson, Margo, Ph.D., M.Sc., B.Sc. (OT), O.T. Reg. (Ont.), F.C.A.O.T.

Dr. Paterson is Professor Emerita in the Queen's University School of Rehabilitation Therapy. Dr. Paterson taught at the graduate and undergraduate levels in the Occupational Therapy and the Rehabilitation Sciences programs. Her scholarly contributions are within the areas of professional practice and theory-practice integration; interprofessional education, care, and practice; clinical reasoning; and qualitative research. She currently teaches a course in *Interdisciplinary Studies in Global Health and Disability* at the Bader International Study Centre, Herstmonceux Castle, Queen's University East Sussex, United Kingdom (www.queensu.ca/bisc). Her administrative roles at Queen's included Director of the Office of Interprofessional Education and Practice in the Faculty of Health Sciences from 2009-2012 as well as former Chair of the Occupational Therapy Program. She was one of the Queen's University co-leads for the Canadian Interprofessional Health Leadership Collaborative project from 2012-2015 (www.cihlc.ca). Dr. Paterson is currently the Executive Director of the Association of Occupational Therapy University Programs, which represents the 14 occupational therapy programs in Canada (www.acotup-acpue.ca). She was awarded the Canadian Association of Occupational Therapy (CAOT) Leadership Award in 2012 and the CAOT Fellowship Award in 2015.

Reed, Emily, RN, MSc, PhD(c)

Emily Reed is a nursing PhD candidate at the University of Western Ontario specializing in health human resources and leadership under the supervision of Dr. Heather Laschinger. Her research interests include health care leadership and management, social capital, positive organizational psychology, workplace health and well-being, and new graduate nurses' transitions to the workplace. Emily currently works as a staff nurse in geriatric rehabilitation and a part-time lecturer at the University of Western Ontario.

Van Dijk, Janice, R.N. M.H.Sc., M.Sc., B.Ed.

Janice Van Dijk RN completed her MHSc Community Health focusing on adult education, program development/evaluation, community nutrition at the University of Toronto; she also holds an MSc Physiology and a BEd in Biology and Chemistry from Western University, London Ontario. Janice has worked in areas of basic and applied research, education and health care. Her recent roles include Interprofessional curriculum developer (online and face-to-face courses), project manager for hospice palliative care collaborative practice health care projects, and consultant on how to improve 24-h health care (community) access using information technology. Currently, Janice was a member of the program development team of the Canadian Interprofessional Health Leadership Collaborative (CIHLC), which she joined in May 2012 as a Research Associate for Queen's University.

INTRODUCTION TO INTERPROFESSIONAL CLIENT-CENTERED COLLABORATIVE PRACTICE – A PRACTICAL PRIMER FOR EDUCATORS IN THE PRACTICE SETTING

This book is designed to capture current thinking about the practice of interprofessional client-centered collaborative practice defined as "a partnership between a team of health providers and a client where the client retains control over his/her care and is provided access to the knowledge and skills of team members to arrive at a realistic team shared plan of care and access to the resources to achieve the plan" (Orchard, 2008). The book is also designed to assist practitioners and continuing health educators to enhance the implementation and demonstration of interprofessional collaboration in all areas of health and social care. Each chapter is focused around fictional, but realistic stories about clients and the health and social challenges they face in their interaction with a collaborative care model.

Each chapter has a unique focus for interprofessional client-centered collaborative practice. The reader will be guided through identification of the issues faced by clients and their families, or caregivers and will be provided with strategies that can be adopted to guide practitioners in addressing each challenge from an interprofessional collaborative perspective. The chapters are intended to provide a 'snapshot in time' of the state of this model of practice. A case will be made for change from current models of practice based on research findings when available or from theoretical perspectives when not. The chapter author(s) will then provide suggestions where further work is needed to gain answers to persistent questions related to the topic.

The authors are all identified 'experts' in the field of interprofessional client-centered collaborative practice and will provide their learned thinking related to each of the chapter topics. It is hoped that others will continue to add knowledge, evidence, and theories to the field in creating enhanced meaning around the care that clients receive in addressing their health and social challenges.

To begin the above discussion the reader will be introduced to a synopsis of the state of client-centered collaborative practice. How it is, or is not being realized from the perspective of clients, their families, and health care providers. We begin our book with the client since much of the current rhetoric and many policy directives from governments advocate for a more active role of clients in their care and for changes to the way care is provided in relation to the impact of care on clients' health outcomes. Although many health care providers purport to focus their care on the client, there is limited evidence to suggest that clients are commonly full members of their health care teams (Martin & Finn, 2011; Gruman, Rovner, French, Jeffress, Sofaer, Shaller, & Prager, 2010). The reader will be challenged to reflect on recent discussions within their own health care provider context that may or may not have included the client's or family's viewpoints as expressed by themselves.

A robust quantity of literature related to client/patient/or person centered care exists and within these papers the predominant focus is on the health care providers' perspectives in the dyadic relationship between patient and health care provider. The role of the client as recipient of care is frequently relegated to that of a responder to questions posed to them, or to decisions that are developed and delivered to the client by the health care provider. Throughout this book we will consistently use the term *'client'* even though the predominant literature labels the recipient of health care services as the *patient* or as in the U.K. *service user*. We believe *client* is a more generic term that addresses both health and social care. A predominant pattern being advocated by health policy makers is the role of clients in their own self-care management (Riegel, Jaarsma, & Strömberg, 2013; Lequerica, Donnell & Tate, 2009; Coulter & Ellins, 2007; Hibbard, Mahoney, Stock & Tusler, 2007). However, there is a paucity of literature that demonstrates research outcomes attributed to interactions between the health care providers and their clients in care planning, implementing and evaluating of the actual care offered. This book attempts to address this gap. In client-centered collaborative practice, it is envisioned that the client is a full member of the team and co-creates his/her own care plan with the health care providers. How is this different from traditional care provision? This will be explored further in Chapter 2.

CONTEXT OF PRACTICE

This is the predominant area in which large health teams' function. If we consider a care unit in a hospital setting the staffing is generally composed of a number of registered nurses and medical residents with internal medicine specialists while physical therapists, occupational therapists, social workers, and dietitians come to the unit in response to 'consultation referrals' by physicians/residents or as part of clinical pathways or care maps. Many of these health care providers function within what is termed a multi-disciplinary model of care while others work in interprofessional teams. According to Cohen and Bailey a team is "a collection of individuals who are **interdependent** in their tasks, who **share responsibility** for outcomes, who see themselves and who are seen by others as an intact social entity embedded in one or more larger social systems, and who **manage their relationships** across boundaries" (1997). In this book when the term 'team' is used we are referring to the above characteristics.

In a multi-disciplinary model of care each health care provider assesses the client on his/her own, and may or may not discuss with each other their individual plans for the patient. Often the only documentation source to other health providers are the notes that their fellow health providers leave in a written or electronic record. This form of care was intended to improve the quality of care outcomes for clients based on the shared knowledge, skills and expertise that a team of cross-disciplinary health providers bring together (Fay, Borrill, Amir, Haward & West, 2006).

Although a multidisciplinary form of team care was advocated by health ministries in the 1980's or even earlier, the evidence for its effectiveness has been mixed (Atwal & Caldwell, 2006; Fleissig, Jenkins, Catt, & Fallowfield, 2006). Staff members' differing perceptions and competence to function as team members and persistent hierarchical relationships in institutional settings have been reported as impediments to its implementation (Atwel & Caldwell, 2006). A further issue was the movement in North America during the 1990s to 'casualize' the health professional workforce leading to the breakup of long standing and highly functional teams. Hence self-learned skills among team members in practice may have persisted in some teams while other teams experienced a loss of such expertise. Overall there has been a lack of attention to developing team working skills across professions in educational programs until recently, which may be influencing the varying level of interprofessional collaboration within hospital-based teams. Hence, there is a continuum of practice from multi-disciplinary to interprofessional collaborative. This book will focus on the latter model.

The reader will be provided with a variety of approaches that can be used to re-energize interprofessional teams to enhance their capacity to collaborate in their own work and to integrate the client and their family or other caregiver into their care.

Interprofessional collaborative practice has both task and relational aspects to its enactment. Frequently health administrators focus on the task aspects of care (e.g., number of steps a client processes through) without a focus on the relational aspects to teamwork (e.g., how team members can communicate across their professions). Gittell, Godfrey, and Thistlethwaite (2013) discuss the need for relational coordination which they define as "a mutually reinforcing process of communicating and relating for the purpose of task integration" (p. 210). Gittell tested a model of service relationship and customer outcomes in a study of 338 health providers and 878 of their clients in in-patient surgical units and found that provider-provider relationships influence client outcomes (2002). She concluded that "effective relationships with the [client] depend, in part, on well-functioning relationships between the service providers who are jointly involved in the delivery of services to that [client]" (Gittell , 2002, p. 308). Thus the need to focus continuing education programs on team work among health providers as a means to improve client outcomes is a key to effective care and we will argue the engagement of and inclusion of the client in shaping their care can further increase improvements in their health outcomes.

However, a lack of attention to the relational development of team members will continue to undermine the effectiveness of any form of teamwork amongst health providers (Carpenter, Schneider, Brandon & Wooff, 2003). Thus moving to interprofessional collaborative practice defined as "a partnership between a team of health providers and a client in a participatory, collaborative and coordinated approach to shared decision- making around health and social issues" (Orchard,Curran, & Kabene, 2005) where all team members are intended to work together in shaping, implementing, and evaluating care for their clients can perhaps be envisioned as a further evolution from multidisciplinary teamwork. Recognition that other health care providers and the client are key elements in effective health service delivery was important. Now we need to focus on how those interdependent parts communicate and co-ordinate information and care in an integrated and seamless fashion.

The challenge for continuing health educators is how to develop strategies and create meaningful learning activities that will attract a cross section of health providers to learn how to work more effectively in collaborative interprofessional teams. Three aspects that can lay a foundation for relational development in teams include: addressing differing perceptions of teamwork, developing consistent levels of skills acquisitions to function as a team member; and addressing power relationships between and among health care providers.

Addressing Differing Perceptions of Teamwork

The development of interprofessional team working skills within pre-licensure programs is a new area of education. Hence, many post-licensure practitioners will not have ecperienced learning in this vital area of practice. Denneskere, Robyns, Vanhaecht, Euwema, Panella, Lodewijckx, Leigheb, Sermeus and the EQCP-study group identified the need to focus on team indicators related to: team context/structure (culture and climate for team of organization; team interdependence; resources; and coordinating mechanisms), team process (team relations; quality of team leadership; team communication; team task/reflexivity; team vision; team orientation; team mental model; and belief in teamwork), and team outcomes (perceive coordination of care processes; team effectiveness; perceive communication with client/family; satisfaction; perceive follow-up of care; and professional agreements on best practices) (Denneskere et al., 2011).

Interprofessional collaborative teamwork training will require consideration of how interprofessional teamwork learning is enacted. There are several ways of doing this. The most common ones are through competencies or capabilities. The Canadian Interprofessional Healthcare Collaborative's (CIHC) National Framework for Interprofessional Collaboration has been designed to focus on the process of IPCP. It incorporates Roegier's integrative pedagogy in which a heath team's shared knowledge, skills, attitudes and values are integrated to arrive at their team judgments around care for their clients and are shaped by Tardiff's characteristics of competence: complexity (dynamic organization of competencies); additive (integration of knowledge, skills, attitudes and values to formulate judgments); integrative (dependent on the shared contributions of the team members); developmental (moves from novice to expert over time); and evolutionary (applied within a given context leading to ongoing new understandings). In the framework the competencies evolve from, and are foundational to, the goal which is interprofessional collaborative practice. There are six: client/family/community centered care; interprofessional communication; role clarification; team functioning; interprofessional conflict resolution and collaborative leadership. Descriptors found in the online downloadable document www.cihc.ca/files/CIHC_IPCOMPETENCIES_Feb1210.pdf. may be used to guide the development of strategies to achieve learning goals in continuing education sessions.

Capabilities for teamwork practice have also been advocated by Walsh, Gordon, Marshall, Wilson and Hunt, (2005) and McNair (2005). Capability is defined as an integrated application of knowledge where the "… practitioner can adapt to change, develop new behaviors and continue to improve performance" (Fraser & Greenhalgh, 2001, p.800) .These authors challenge the use of competencies as too limiting in practice given the complexity of clients. The former authors suggest there are four domains of capabilities: ethical practice, knowledge in practice, interprofessional working, and reflection Walsh et al., 2005) while the latter author expands the domains to five and includes values and changes interprofessional working to skills for the process of care and changes reflection to application (McNair, 2005). Other authors suggest that capabilities are simply a form of competence (Garavan, & McGuire, 2001). Chapter 1 will provide a more in depth discussion of the debates around competence, competencies, and capabilities in practice.

Developing Consistent Levels of Skills Acquisition to Function As a Team Member

In order to understand how to focus continuing education towards consistent team member functioning we need to reflect on how health providers are socialized and educated to enact their roles.

Professional Socialization

Life experiences shape our perceptions about the roles of health professionals. These experiences are influenced by societal imaging of professionals often through media. These sources shape images of a future professional identity and influence goal setting to become that professional as compared to other professionals. These images and perceptions have both accurate and inaccurate views about their chosen and other professionals. When an individual is successful in gaining admission into a health professional educational program faculty re-shape the student to envision their own accurate professional identity but, until recently, did not guide the student to also gain an accurate understanding of other professionals roles they will be working with. Once professional identities are established they are resistant to change based on what Shulman terms a profession's signature pedagogy (2005). Shulman sees the enactment of our professional practice as creating the dimensions of our professional work or socialization. As you reflect on your own practice and how do you uniquely think within your professional role? How accurate is our understanding of the role of other health professionals with whom you work?

Uni-Disciplinary Education

Professional identities evolve through a system of education in which professionals learn their 'craft' within their own professional grouping, this is termed uni-disciplinary education. Such an approach creates a strong affinity for learners to own professional group (termed the in-group) and a level of disaffection with other health professionals (the out-group) (Pettigrew & Troop, 2008). Without attention to learning more about other professionals to decrease misperceptions about them, a level of distrust and perceptions of varying values of each other continues within teams and is detrimental to development of collaborative teamwork.

It would appear that the more health providers learn about each other's roles, knowledge, skills, and expertise (learning about the outgroup) the greater the likelihood of their willing to move out of their profession-specific in-group (changing behavior) and moving towards a shared interprofessional in-group (generating affective ties). Pettigrew and Troop studied three mediators to the above and found that *reduction of anxiety in an outgroup* member joining an in-group was needed initially, followed by developing *empathy from both in-group and outgroup members* towards each other and finally gaining *clarity around the roles of* each member is necessary to support intergroup contact (2008) and collaborative teamwork. As you read the chapters in this book you are encouraged to consider how socialization and professional education may be influencing the practice within each topic area.

Addressing Power Relationships between Health Provider Groups

The persistence of status differences within the health system continue to influence whose decision making is authorized and valued. This is seen by several authors as problematic to effective multidisciplinary and interprofessional collaborative teamwork (Gair & Hartley, 2001; Coombs, & Ersser, 2004; Nugus, Greefield, Travaglia, Westbrook & Braithwaite, 2010). At the same time when teams focused on key clusters of clients, such as those in geriatric or mental health units, more shared teamwork was observed (Gair & Hartey, 2001). They attributed this finding to the length of time on the team and also the stability of the team. These factors seemed to create a team environment where trust and openness to hearing other viewpoints could be accepted (Gair & Hartey, 2001). Nugus et al., found that competitive (dominance of one health provider over another) and collaborative power (enacted both role distinctiveness and interchangeability) were exercised within teams and that individuals demonstrated unconsciously both benevolence and mutual empathy for team members. Hence, power relationships are a continuing reality of the institutional environment (Nugus, et al., 2010). Power relationships can be enacted by any professional within a team through exercising control over others. Continuing education sessions in which a trusting environment is fostered between parties and all participants show a willingness to listen opening and carefully to each other may create learning settings to address this persistent issue.

CLIENT INVOLVEMENT IN THEIR CARE

We began this introduction with a definition of interprofessional client-centered collaborative practice but a great deal of the discussion has been health professional in team specific. We assert what is missing from the literature then is the inclusion of the client and family as members of the collaborative team. The heath provider driven approach to care delivery is still predominated by their evidence and experiential based perceptions of care needs of clients and individual viewpoints on what these needs are still predominates care. If we consider how client involvement is envisioned in the current health system through both multidisciplinary and interprofessional collaborative teams, the client role shows limited change. There is a growing emphasis on the importance of the client having a 'voice' in their care which has been directed through some government Acts such as the NHS and Community Care Act 1991 in the U.K., and the Excellent Care for All Act in the province of Ontario, Canada. Studies of the UK implementation of clients' service user involvement in an ethnography of institutional programs for Stroke clients by Fudge, Wolfe and McKevitt found "health care professionals and service users understand and practice user involvement in different sways according to individual ideologies, circumstances, and needs" (2007, p.1). Service user involvement seems to be related to the beliefs held by health providers as to the role and value of clients in their involvement. There are no published studies related to enactment of the Ontario Act to date that can help in further understanding of the client role.

In other literature cited health professionals exhibit a level of comfort in clients being involved at health policy and health program levels. However, there is a reticence for client involvement within their health care teams – this discomfort seems to be attributed to a misunderstanding of the value of client contributions into health teams by sharing how they manage their care and concurrently listening to and responding to suggested approaches to their care provided by a variety of health providers that can create greater efficiency in care planning and a greater likelihood of the client embracing and completing the care the team (including the client) arrives at from such discussions. It is this 'living expert' role that needs to be understood and welcomed by health providers for client-centered collaborative practice to be enacted. As the reader moves through this book's chapters you will be provided with insights on how to attend to client inclusion that is based on their voice and expressed needs from the health providers.

In summary organizational psychologists are noting the need to focus on relationship building to develop a workforce which can be responsive to the changing needs of clients and their health needs. Thus, there seems to be a misfit between hospital administrative practices, and the needs for service provision for particularly clients with complex needs who have the potential to disproportionately utilize higher health services from the norm of the population. Thus a re-focus on the relationship building between health providers and between them and their clients and families that is interprofessional client-centered collaborative practice to overcome the time and workload wasters that arise from current practices.

The argument we raise in this book is the need to re-focus our health providers towards interprofessional client/family-centered collaborative practice. An approach to care that creates more than simple engagement of clients in their care, but to a partnership between health providers and clients with their families to create shared plans of care that fit within the lifestyle and capacity of these parties and within the resources of the systems.

To achieve such a model of care cannot occur with directing attention to the preparation of health providers to practice within such relational associations. Accomplishing this shift in practice necessitates an understanding of what is our socialization into health provider roles, and how our education structures transformed into the health providers we currently are in the health systems today. Then to consider the fit between the above and the current needs of our clients and the characteristics of the health system operation today. Such an understanding has the potential to help each health provider to challenge their existing assumptions and consider potential new thinking to fit within the changing needs of clients and our populations. We argue this to be interprofessional client/family-centered collaborative practice.

OVERVIEW OF BOOK CHAPTERS

Each chapter in this book will assist in identifying some challenges and strategies to overcome professional silos and to assist learners to gain insight into how learning about each other and working together can be a benefit to themselves, their clients, and their organizations. Hence it will focus on contexts for practice and will focus on approaches that have been shown to be successful, and will then suggest areas for further study needed to achieve robust evidence of IPC effectiveness in practice.

In chapter 1 we focus on issues associated with competence to practice within an interprofessional client-centered perspective and then in chapter 2 we offer a discussion of a framework for interprofessional client-centered collaborative practice. Chapter 3 introduces perioperative practice within the context of interprofessional client-centered collaborative practice which is followed by the discussion of the individual health professional's role within a team in this context of practice. In Chapter 4 discussions focus on mental health recovery in community settings and the roles of team members with their clients while in chapter 5 the focus is on the how to embed mental health recovery into practice settings. Chapter 6 provides a discussion on how to shift the culture in organizations to embrace interprofessional education and collaborative practice. Chapter 7 explores how to engage physicians in continuing interprofessional development. In chapter 8 a discussion on workplace environments needed for interprofessional client-centered collaborative practice to be realized is provided. While in Chapter 9 provides a discussion on whether collaborative practice can have an impact on patient safety. In chapter 10 the reader will be provided with an overview of how health teams can provide interprofessional collaborative practice in primary health care and this is followed by addressing theory into practice when running interprofessional health clinics in chapter 11. Discussion about how to evaluate practice programs using a logic framework analysis model. In the final chapter a discussion of measurement for interprofessional client-centered collaborative practice is provided in which assessment of performance of the individual in a team and the total team are explored.

REFERENCES

Atwal, A., & Caldwell, K., (2006). Nurses' perceptions of multidisciplinary team work in acute health-care. *International Journal of Nursing Practice, 12*, 359-365. DOI: 10.1111lj.1440-172x.2006.00595.x.

Canadian Interprofessional Healthcare Collaborative (2010*). The CIHC National interprofessional collaboration competency framework*. Vancouver: CIHC.

Carpenter, J., Schneider, J., Brandon, r., & Wooff, D. (2003). Working in multidisciplinary community mental health teams: the impact on social workers and health professionals of integrated mental health care. *British Journal of Social Work, 33*(8), 1081-1103.

Coombs, M., & Ersser, S.J., (2004). Medical hegemony in decision-making – a barrier to interdisciplinary working in intensive care? *Journal of Advanced Nursing, 46*(3), 245-252.

Coulter, A. (2007). Effectiveness of strategies of informing, educating, and involving patients. *British Medical Journal, 335*(July), 24-27

Deneckere, S., Robyns, N., Vanhaecht, K., Euwema, M., Panella, M., Lodewijckx, C., Leigheb, F., & Sermeus, W. (2011). Indicators for follow-up of multidisciplinary teamwork in care processes: Results of an international expert panel. *Evaluation and the Health Professions, 34*(3), 258-277. DOI: 10.1177/0163278710393736.

Fay, D., Borrill, C., Amir, S., Howard, R., & West, M.A. (2006). Getting the most out of multidisciplinary teams: A multi-sample study of team innovation in health care. *Journal of Occupational and Organizational Psychology, 79*, 553-567. DOI: 10.1348/096317905X72128.

Fleissig, A., Jenkins, V., Catt, S., & Fallowfield, L. (2006). Multidisciplinary teams in cancer care: are they effective in the UK? *Lancet Oncology, 7*, 935-43.

Fraser, S.W., & Greenhalgh, T. (2001). Complexity science: Coping with complexity: Educating for capability. *British Medical Journal, 323*(7316), 799-803.

Fudge, N., Wolfe, C.D.A., & McKevitt, C. (2007). Assessing the promise of user involvement in health service development: ethnographic study. British Medical Journal, ONLINE FIRST, 1-8. DOI: 10.1136/bmj.39456.662257.BE.

Gair, G.., & Hartery, T., (2001). Medical dominance in multidisciplinary teamwork: A case study of discharge decision-making in a geriatric assessment unit. Journal of Nursing Management, 9, 3-11

Garavan, T.N., & McGuire, D., (2001). Competencies and workplace learning: some reflections on the rhetoric and the reality. *Journal of Workplace Learning, 13*(4), 144-164. DOI: 10.1108/13665620110391097.

Gittell, J.H., Godfrey, M. and Thistlethwaite, J. (2013). Interprofessional collaborative practice and relational coordination: Improving healthcare through relationships. *Journal of Interprofessional Care, 27*:210-13. DOI: 10.3109/13561820.2012.73056

Gruman, J., Rovner, M.H., French, M.E., Jeffress, D., Sofaer, S., shaller, D., & Prager, D.J. (2010). From patient education to patient engagement: Implications for the field of patient education. *Patient Education & Counseling, 78*, 350-356. DOI: 10.1016/j.pec.2010.02.002.

Hibbard, J.H., Mahoney, E.R., Stock, R., & Tusler, (2007). Self-management and health care utilization. *Health Services Research, 42*(4), 1443-1463. DOI: 10.1111/j.1475-6773.2006.00669x.

Lequerica, A.H., Donnell, C.S., & Tate, D.G., (2009). Patient engagement in rehabilitation therapy: physical and occupational therapist impressions. *Disability and Rehabilitation, 31*(9), 753-760. DOI: 10.1080/09638280802309095.

Martin, G.P., & Finn, R. (2011). Patients as team members: opportunities, challenges and paradoxes of including patients in multi-professional healthcare teams. *Sociology of Health & Illness, 33*(7), 1050-1065. DOI: 10.1111/j.1467-9566.2011.01356.x.

McNair, R.P. (2005). The case for educating health care students in professionalism as the core content of interprofessional education. *Medical Education, 39*, 456-464. DOI: 10.1111/.1365-2929.2005.02116.x.

Nugus, P., Greenfield, D., Tavaglia, J., Westbrook, J., & Braithwaite. (2010). How and where clinicians exercise power: interprofessional relations in health care. *Social Science & Medicine, 71*, 898-909. DOI 10.1016/j.socscimed.2010.05.029.

Pettigrew, T.F., & Tropp, L.R. (2008). How does intergroup contact reduce prejudice: Meta-analytic tests of three mediators. *European Journal of Social Psychology, 38*, 922-934. DOI 10.1002/ejsp.504.

Orchard, C.A. (2008). *Patient centred collaborative care.* Canadian Health Services Research Foundation, http://youtube/h7jHp5ooNec

Orchard CA, Curran V, Kabene S. (2005). Creating a culture of interdisciplinary collaborative professional practice. *Med Education Online [serial online],10*:11. Available from http://www.med-ed-online.org

Riegel, B., Jaarsma, T., & Strömberg, A. (2012). A middle-range theory of self-care of chronic illness. *Advances in Nursing Science, 35*(3), 194-204. DOI: 10.1097/ANS.0b013e318261b1ba.

Shulman, A.S. (2005). Signature Pedagogies in the professions. Daedalus, 134(3), 52-59.

Walsh, C.L., Gordon, M.F., Marshall, M., Wilson, F., & Hunt, T. (2005). Interprofessional capability: A developing framework for interprofessional education. *Nursing Education in Practice, 5*, 230-237. DOI: 10.1016/j.nepr.2004.12.004.

In: Interprofessional Client-Centred Collaborative Practice   ISBN: 978-1-63483-754-5
Editor: Carole Orchard   © 2015 Nova Science Publishers, Inc.

Chapter 1

TOWARDS A FRAMEWORK OF CLIENT-CENTERED COLLABORATIVE PRACTICE

Carole Orchard
Western University, London, ON, Canada

ABSTRACT

The chapter opens with a discussion on the growing impact of chronic disease in populations and the health system pressures to meet demands for ongoing care. In response a focus has shifted to delivery of care through teamwork, advocated because of the burgeoning health human resource shortages. The focus then shifts to how a framework for client-centered collaborative practice can be created in which a partnering relationship develops between clients, their families, and health providers within interprofessional teams. Exploration of this framework begins with a discussion about client engagement and client participation with the role of clients in their self-care being presented as a shift in traditional care provision. A discussion is then presented on the partnering relationships between clients and health providers in which they work together to achieve a common goal through non-hierarchical interactions and combining of their shared resources used through mutual respect for each other's skills and competences as well as shared decision-making leading towards set goals. A case study is provided to operationalize the above concepts. Finally, collaborative client-centered care is provided as the outcome of all parties negotiating and adapting individual inputs into options for care to arrive at a shared plan all can support.

Keywords: Client engagement, client participation, shared decision-making, client centered

INTRODUCTION

A great deal of rhetoric has been evident around client-centered practice with limited evidence of its enactment within interprofessional teams, yet in health care systems many institutions have included a focus on client-centered care in their mission statements. In addition, continuing education programs rarely integrate the perspective of the client and family as key facilitators of practice-based learning. Although much has been touted about the importance of client involvement in their care, practice models continue to advocate existing professional and interprofessional foci, rarely including client and family members as part of the model or, indeed, as key partners in care decisions.

Current multi-disciplinary and teamwork models continue to reinforce profession-specific foci leading to unique language, communication patterns, approaches to client encounters, and ethical codes generated within professions. These are often developed in isolation from those who are the focus of practice outcomes, namely the clients and their families or carers. These practices continue to support health professionals as 'experts,' creating power differentials between providers and clients, while mission and vision statements place clients at the center of their care. Up to one-third of the world's population now experience chronic diseases. While no new data have been made easily available, the World Health Organization (WHO) reported in 2014 that "four chronic diseases (cardiovascular, cancer, chronic respiratory, and diabetes) are responsible for 82% of the mortality rates worldwide" (p. xi.) and further that "the number of NCD [non-communicable or chronic disease] deaths has increased worldwide and in every region since 2000" (p. 9). To address a reduction in the loss of productivity and quality of life for those with these diseases, WHO recommends that health systems "identify and address health-system barriers to NCD [non-communicable or chronic disease] care, with a special focus on strengthening patient centered primary health care" (World Health Organization, 2014, p. 127). The growing prevalence of chronic diseases are reflective of improved treatment and pharmacological advances, leading to increased life expectancy and improved function and quality of life for those with a chronic disease or injury. However, our health systems are often focused solely on acute illness while only recently advocating for the adoption of healthy lifestyles, which in many countries and cases may be beyond the reach (e.g., those who are below the poverty level). The concerns about health system costs have caused governments to adopt policy directives that push management of their care to the patient, particularly for those with chronic diseases that necessitated ongoing monitoring. As limited health human resources are available and accessible to patients, the need increases to have models of care that provide a means to support the health requirements of more and more complex patients while helping these same patients to manage their own ongoing care within their capacities within their home communities. Interprofessional patient-centered collaborative practice is such a model. However, enacting this form of practice necessitates a shift in how patients and their families see their roles in managing, monitoring, and maintaining their health states and a shift in the assumptions health professionals hold about the role of clients managing their care, with themselves as facilitators and supporters or coaches for these clients. This is of particular importance when patients or clients are in this role in models such as mid-range theory of self-care management in chronic diseases (Riegel, Jaarsma, & Strömberg, 2012) and when conducting assessments of their ability to care for themselves through such instruments as the Illness Perception Questionnaire (Moss-Morris et al., 2002).

In this chapter we will review the existing literature related to interprofessional teamwork and client engagement or participation in their care. This will be followed by a discussion of the role of evidence-informed practice within an interprofessional collaborative team, and finally how all these elements can be brought together into an integrated practice framework. The framework will then be applied into a case situation to demonstrate how a continuing interprofessional educator might develop the means to begin influencing a broader shift from the traditional focus on the individualized health provider to all-party participation in shared care around shared goals with the inclusion of patients and family members.

CLIENT ENGAGEMENT

Client engagement is a popular term used by health system policymakers and administrators to describe a direction for inclusion of the client and family or carer in influencing services and care provided that reflects their needs, preferences, and choices. Engagement has been defined as "actions people take for their health and to benefit from health care" (Carman et al., 2013, p. 223). However, a disconnection remains between the definition, its theoretical foundation, actual practice, and furthermore to the dimensions of what fosters client engagement (Barello, Graffigna, & Vegni, 2012, p. 1). Carman et al., (2013) suggested that client engagement is characterized by four features: (a) shared power and responsibility, (b) clients as active partners in defining agendas (in policy and in program committee work), or making decisions (when at the direct care interface level), (c) provision of bidirectional information flows throughout the process, and (d) sharing in decision-making responsibility. They further provided a framework arguing that client engagement is positioned on a continuum from consultation to involvement and finally to partnership and shared leadership (Carman et al., 2013). Engagement can occur at three different levels within organizations — at the policymaking level, the organizational design and governance level, and the direct-care level (Carman et al., 2013).

It is now becoming more common to find clients and family members on quality improvement committees and for health agencies to authentically implement client and family advisory committees. Clients and family members have also increasingly been invited to participate at the policy level by governments. This participation is an outcome of legislation found in the United Kingdom, Australia, New Zealand, and in the provinces of British Columbia and Ontario in Canada. Hence, the engagement of clients is becoming an expectation within health systems. However, the inclusion of clients and their family members at the direct-care level is, as Haigh (2008) suggested, "patchy" (p. 458) and "superficial" (p. 458). Clancy (2011) further cautioned, "Well-intended initiatives often appear to fall short of collective aspirations that build a system responsible to the needs of patients and families" (p. 390). In order to move to greater authentic inclusion of clients and their chosen caregivers as active participants in their care requires supportive environments created at health institutional governance levels. To do so will require the "embracing of new norms and substantial changes to their culture, processes, and structure" (Carman et al., 2013, p. 228).

Currently, most health institutions tend to be system focused. They may have a stated value of being client-centered; however, the processing of clients through their institutions is rarely designed around comprehensive client-centered care, but rather the client is required to fit into the service structures, processes, and schedules of the institution. A further constraint for many clients with chronic disease is the acute focus of care within many hospitals. This means that clients with chronic diseases are left to acquire an acute complication of their disease before health services and those professionals working in these agencies provide care to these clients. Thus, many clients are left to carry out their own self-care following the resolution of a complication. However, these clients have asked for monitoring programs to guide and to support them as they manage their own health state to prevent complications. Interestingly, in a time of financial constraints one would expect that health agencies would quickly re-focus their efforts around such support to save costs associated with more expensive treatment for complications. An example is the lack of ongoing support programs to assist clients with diabetes to manage, monitor, and maintain their health. In another example, renal failure as an outcome of diabetes is preventable with good long-term management. When renal failure arises as a complication it requires the most expensive treatment through provision of ongoing dialysis care. Does it not make sense to re-think care approaches to address such outcomes and prevent them? Such an intervention would decrease health care costs and the use of resources while also providing a higher quality of life for those with diabetes. This means that health care teams need to develop ongoing monitoring approaches to assist in partnerships with these clients to maintain their health related to their diet, exercise, medication regime, and so forth. Thus, an interprofessional team is needed to ensure the comprehensive nature of care is addressed in those clients with complex chronic diseases such as diabetes.

A shift is thus required from what is termed traditional care (Sahlsten, Larsson, Sjöström, & Plos, 2009) or also referred to as older paternalistic paradigms (Carman et al., 2013). In such forms of practice the assumption is "that ... [health providers] know best, [and should] make decisions on behalf of clients without involving them" (Coulter, 1999, p. 719). In true client engagement there is a shift to a focus on "inclusion of patients and family members in all aspects of care delivery and design" (Gittell, Godfrey, & Thistlethwaite, 2013, p. 211). Engaging clients in learning that helps assist them in their own self-management is likely to result in more effective use of resources with a concomitant reduction in overall health costs (Barello et al., 2012).

How can we transform belief systems to adopt client engagement in their care? Shifts are needed beyond just administrators and policymakers to health providers, clients, and their family members or chosen caregivers. Health professionals who persist in caring for their clients using a non-collaborative approach have the potential to provide care that is professional specific in a time when interprofessional teamwork is required. Hindrances have been identified as to why health providers are reluctant to shift into collaborative models of care with their clients; these include health care providers' perceptions that (a) clients lack sufficient knowledge and understanding to participate (Henderson, 2003); (b) they need to hold on to power and control to support their beliefs that they know best for clients (Henderson, 2003); (c) clients should trust that health providers to know best (Saunders, 1995); (d) such care will increase demands by clients for more care (Saunders, 1995); (e) their role will be undermined (Saunders, 1995); and (f) submissive care to clients can be provided faster and safer (Saunders, 1995). If we analyzed these hindrances, most reside within health providers and their views of what they would be giving up — power, control, expertise — undermining of their professional role. The other hindrances cited related to client knowledge and higher demands for services. The former issue can be addressed by understanding clients' knowledge needs and addressing these, while the latter is a difficult argument to accept. If clients were able to monitor their chronic condition and thus minimize complications it would seem that they would require fewer health system resources rather than more. Thus, it is difficult to accept the identified 'hindrances' beyond that of a resistance to change due to the loss of professional status, power, and control over clients.

In a Cochrane review of patient engagement, Gruman et al., (2010) found, "Most well-developed interventions to increase engagement are directed at modifying patient medical compliance, chronic disease self-management and transitional behaviors associated with promotion of health and prevention of disease, smoking, diet and exercise" (p. 354). A further finding was "the stifling effect that health professionals appear to have upon the voice of service users [patients] and providers" (Haigh, 2008, p. 458). Further evidence of the often-existing power differential between health providers and clients was found in a qualitative study by Frank, Asp, and Dahlberg (2008) who focused on client participation in emergency care. Frank et al., identified three themes that related to patient participation in their care: caregivers offer conditional participation, patients demand participation, and mutual participation. They concluded that "the conceptualization of patient participation is consequently conditional and on the caregivers' conditions" (Frank et al., 2008, p. 2560). In a further grounded theory study, Sahlsten et al., (2009) identified the core category as being insight through consideration that is dependent on providing an obliging atmosphere and emotional responses that are sensitive, thoughtful, and trustworthy between parties through a dialogic process that supports learning between the parties and results in gaining competence in partnering within a supportive environment. Sahlsten et al., (2009) concluded, "The present findings imply that nurses ought to change their traditional role from being a giver and helper to instead guiding and providing the patients with opportunities to take more control over their own situation" (p. 495). The same message is likely to apply to other health provider groups as well. Shifting to a truly client- and family-centered care approach requires, as one practitioner stated to me, "not a change in how we practice, but a change in how we think about our practice" (Clinical Psychologist, personal communication, March 20th, 2009).

It appears that collaborative practice necessitates health providers to give up aspects of their controlling role while having clients 'stretch' their previous participation in their care. Clancy (2011) suggested that for health providers to shift to more collaborative care clients, must meet a set of expectations, including whether and when to seek care; which plans and providers meet their needs; how to manage their health; and how to cope with sometimes conflicting advice from providers, friends, and family. Coulter (2012) shifted the expectations to what clients want from health providers, and specifically noted the following client desires:

> [The] ability to access timely, reliable, effective, and safe health care when ... [needed];
> ... adequate information and support to participate in decisions that affect them; ... [be treated with] empathy, dignity, and respect; ... told about options for treating or managing their condition and that their preferences ... [are then taken] into account; and ... not .. [having] to worry about the financial consequences of being ill. (p. 80)

Some authors have suggested stretching clients' participation to demonstrate this new role in the team. However, there is a paucity of writing on what this team role is for clients. What is provided relates to the role of clients in their own care, excluding the interconnection between their role and that of the interprofessional collaborative team.

What about the client and family? They too have roles that require a shift in their view of the health provider/client/family interactions. What might that role look like? An example of a potential description is provided below.

Who Is a Patient or Client?

The University of Western Ontario, Office of the Interprofessional Health Education & Research (2015) provided the following definition of a patient or client: "An individual who seeks help to manage a health and/or social issue(s) that is (are) interfering with his/her desired capacity to fully participate in his/her family and community" ("Who is a Patient," para. 1).

What Can the Patient or Client do in a Team?

The University of Western Ontario, Office of the Interprofessional Health Education & Research (2015) described the role of the patient or client within the interprofessional care team:

> The patient/client expresses her/his lived experience of illness or injury and conveys what their own values and priorities are. This "story" (as told by the patient) is critical to the team's understanding of the patient/client and to developing appropriate goals and care plan. The patient/client brings into a health and social care team how his/her daily life is impacted by their health and/or social issues (and vice versa) and how suggested treatments and/or actions from the team can be adapted (or not) into their activities of daily living. ("What Can the Patient," para. 1)

How Does the Patient or Client Fit into a Team?

The following excerpt depicts how the patient fits in to the interprofessional care team:

> The patient/client becomes a true member of the interprofessional patient/client centred team in which he/she retains control over his/her care and is provided with the knowledge, skills, and expertise of the health/social care providers so that a plan of care can be negotiated within existing resources. (University of Western Ontario, Office of the Interprofessional Health Education & Research, 2015, "How does the Patient," para. 1)

Education and Preparation

In discussing preparation and education regarding collaborating within a health care team, the University of Western Ontario, Office of the Interprofessional Health Education & Research (2015) stated,

> The patient/client brings his/her understanding of health and social needs and ensures these are recognized within his/her own frame of reference in the interaction with health and social care providers to assist in shaping a plan to address, monitor and reduce/resolve the identified issues. As a patient/client you seek to learn how to prepare yourself to be involved as a team member in your care. ("Education," para. 1)

The Patient or Client Connecting to a Collaborative Practice Model

At the health care team level, the patient or client can request the following:

1. all needed health and social care providers meet with you at the same time to coordinate your care,
2. health and social care providers give you as the patient/client an equal voice in discussions around your care,
3. health and social care providers be willing to negotiate care with you to fit in with what is feasible in your life and to support a reduction/resolution of your health/social issues,
4. the community providers necessary to continue to support your care can be part of the team, and know the needs and plan developed between you and all the health/social care providers to ensure continuance of the plan through a seamless transition from one level of care to another (e.g., hospital to home). (University of Western Ontario, Office of the Interprofessional Health Education & Research, 2015, "Patient/Client Connecting," para. 5–8)

Discussions are now emerging around how this role might be actualized. Coulter (2012) suggested that the goal of client engagement is "to support and strengthen patients' determination of their health care needs and self-care efforts with a view to obtaining maximum value and improved health outcomes" (p. 81). What is proposed in the above discussion is not the norm of a role that patients or clients expect to assume with their health providers in many health settings at the present time. The literature does support positive outcomes from such involvement; clients experience greater care satisfaction, decrease nosocomial infections, decreased falls, and shortened lengths of hospital stays, and health providers experience greater job satisfaction and decreased turnover. There is limited literature to date discussing the role of the patient or client within interprofessional collaborative teams.

Most of the literature has focused on single dyadic interactions between clients and one health provider. However, recent literature and studies are beginning to focus on the elements, conditions, and attitudes needed for this shift to occur within both health providers and clients. Determining what preparation clients require to be able to participate in collaborative teams is scant. A study by Martin (2011) focused on the success of client engagement at a program level in the United Kingdom. He found that success in their team role was dependent on their feelings of being known within the group, and also being given a clearly stated and supported role in the team. Hence, health care institutions likely require orientation programs to be in place that assist clients in assuming their role. When a client is unable to assume such a role due to his or her condition, the role may be transferred to a chosen caregiver who may be a relative or friend. Maintaining the current belief that health providers can assume the client's role in representing client needs is likely to perpetuate a paternalistic approach to care. We will explore what content is required in such an orientation in the next section of this chapter.

CLIENT PARTICIPATION

There is a difference between client engagement and client participation; in the former there is an effort to bring clients and health providers together to work in partnerships, while in the latter client participation relates to the actions taken to realize these partnerships. The client's level of participation is reported to be dependent on "how much information flows between patient and provider; how active a role the patient has in care decisions; [and] how involved the patient ... becomes [in his or her care]" (Carman et al., 2013, p. 219). However, to date, as Coulter (1999) noted, there is a paucity of research to understand clients' willingness to assume a decision-making responsibility within partnerships. Two aspects associated with this participation have been studied: client health literacy and client activation.

Client Health Literacy

A great deal of, perhaps biased, perspectives have long been associated with the thorny issue of who will or will not be active with their care. Coulter (2012) believes that for clients to participate in their care requires them to be able to read literature about their condition, understand what they are reading, and be able to act on the information they have understood. Health literacy is also believed to be a moderator for clients' health outcomes (Lee, Arozullah, & Cho, 2004). Health providers as a rule have achieved at least procedural knowing and many function using constructed knowing. Unless they have gained an understanding of how to adapt their interactions with clients within the client's capacity to understand and process information there is a strong likelihood that helping a client towards more participation in her or his care will be ineffective. Thus, critiques of studies showing education, health literacy, age, and so forth as indicators of participation may be remiss in not attending to how health providers adapt their interactions with clients considering their health literacy. When these are controlled for, will the same results be found? Studies are needed to focus on this important area.

Client–Health Provider Relationships

What is known about client activation? Sahlsten, Larsson, Sjöström, and Plos (2008) carried out a concept analysis of client activation and identified three clusters of their choices for participation: (a) "express their views and opinions or state their preferences without prompting" (p. 5), (b) "express their views and opinions or state their preferences when invited to do [so]" (p. 6), or (c) "accepts the decisions that are made" (p. 5). Features that are reported to be associated with client participation include having an established relationship between patients and health providers; surrendering of some power or control to clients by health providers; clients and health providers sharing of information and knowledge; and active mutual engagement in intellectual or physical activities (or both) between clients and health providers (Sahlsten et al., 2008). However, these attributes do not address the importance of understanding and processing information in allowing these attributes to be realized. Other writers have suggested the use of relationship-centered care, defined as "care in which all participants appreciate the importance of their relationships with one another" (Beach & Inui, 2006, p. S3) as a means to support more patient activation. Relationship-centered care is comprised of four principles for building relationships: (a) a focus on the "personhood of the participants" (Beach & Inui, 2006, p. S3); (b) attention to "affect and emotion [as] important components of these relationships" (p. S3); (c) "relationships occur[ing] in the context of reciprocal influence" (p. S3); and (d) "formation and maintenance of genuine relationships" (p. S3).

However, in all these pronouncements about relationship building the voice of the client and family appear to be absent. While relationship building is associated with trust, gaining trust necessitates all parties valuing each other's competence and abilities. This valuing allows the participants to enter into conditional relationships. If health providers do not perceive clients to be competent in their knowledge and skills to manage their own care, how does this impact on the ability of these relationships being established and supported? Furthermore, if relationships take time to develop, how can short office-based visits (often a reality in primary care environments) result in development of trust between clients and health providers? Coulter (2012) suggests, "If patients are to play a more effective role [in their care] they must be better supported, be better informed, be more discriminating about the effects of medical treatment, and have more opportunities for participation" (p. 81). Furthermore, Carman et al., (2013) suggest that for true partnerships (the outcome of relationship development and coordination across all parties) to be enacted clients and health providers need to work together to achieve a common goal, share mutual respect for each other's skills and competences through non-hierarchical interactions, and share in decision-making and responsibility based on recognition that combining their resources has greater benefits in moving towards goals. Hence, clients need clarity about their 'new' role within collaborative teams and how their health providers will exercise their roles. Clients need to communicate with health providers about their health situation, understand the risks and benefits associated with their care choices, ask questions, and access and help develop and update their health record (Carman et al., 2013). In exchange, health providers in collaborative relationships are expected to give timely, complete, and understandable information while eliciting clients' values, beliefs, and tolerance for risks regarding care choices. Collaborative health providers are also expected to give clients encouragement and support and involve their family members and caregivers based on clients' wishes within their teams (Carman et al., 2013, p. 225). To achieve participatory models for care, health providers must give up their power and influence over clients (Carman et al., 2013) and abandon their traditional directive and paternalistic roles (Longtin et al., 2010), and clients must be ready to assume a decision-making responsibility in their care (Coulter, 1999). Clearly the capacity of clients to take risks in sharing their perceived knowledge and skills in managing their health conditions may not be within all clients' capacities to enter into such partnering relationships. Research is needed to determine what factors influence such capacity development and enactment, and to further determine if such models of care result in improvements in clients' health outcomes.

In collaborative client-centered practice health providers become facilitators and coaches to clients. At the same time health providers are still responsible for sharing the best evidence they have about the care needs of clients. However, clients have the right to accept or reject suggestions. Some literature advocates this process gives clients choices. However, it is not free choice, as the term choice implies – it is choice within a set of safe parameters such as best-practice guidelines, clinical evidence, and so forth. For collaborative health providers, this shift in their roles may be seen as incompatible with their perception of safe client care. However, is it truly an issue of safe client care or a reluctance to transfer some responsibility to clients to select from a set of presented options? When clients choose an option that is less acceptable to health providers, is this then labeled as 'unsafe' because it is not the ideal choice deemed by the care provider?

Frank et al., (2008) also identified some conditions required for mutual participation in collaborative relationships to occur. These being sufficient time to engage with clients, having a genuine interest on the part of the caregiver to enter into discussion with clients, and organizations providing opportunity and space to support mutual cooperation (Frank et al., 2008, p. 2559).

Client Activation

Another move to assist in understanding the role of clients in their care and its relationship to their role within collaborative teams relates to work by Hibbard, Mahoney, Stock, and Tusler (2007), who focused on patients' activation to participate in their own self-care management based on decisional theory. Hibbard et al., identified four developmental levels of activation that patients can assume:

1. Passive – clients lack understanding of their role in caring for themselves and expect others to provide their care.
2. Passive – clients either lack basic knowledge and skills needed to provide care for themselves or are unable to connect application of their knowledge and skills to their care.
3. Active – clients have the knowledge to care for themselves and begin to take action, but may lack confidence and skill building to take care of themselves.
4. Active – clients have the knowledge, skills, and confidence to take care of themselves, but may need support if complications or other crises.

These activation levels will influence both the confidence and willingness of clients to participate in their own care with their health provider teams. Knowing a client's level of activation can be assessed by using Hibbard et al.'s Patient Activation Measure.

Relational building between clients and health providers necessitates the ability to listen and to communicate effectively between all team members (including clients and their family members or caregivers) to ensure a shared understanding of the impact of health challenges to clients and their family members. Due to the potential for varying levels of knowing between parties, it is essential that all health providers verify understanding with their clients and family members or chosen caregivers. No longer should health providers assume directive clinical treatment control over clients and their care in the absence of understanding the impacts of treatments to the norm of living of clients. No longer should health providers only focus on clinical treatments based on best practices and evidence without interpreting these into the context and life skills of clients. No longer should health team members be meeting to develop, plan, and implement care without participation of clients who are the implementer and recipient of this care plan. No longer should clients only be allowed to make decisions related to their care from a health provider driven pre-selected group of options (Tomson, Murtagh, & Khaw, 2005). Hence, moving toward client participation in their care requires a sharing of decision-making power between health providers and clients (Sahlsten et al., 2008, p. 5), providing a willingness to persuade each other to modify varying perspectives on treatment decisions through negotiation and adaptation (Abma & Broerse, 2010). Collaborative client-centered care is the outcome of all parties negotiating and adapting individual inputs into options for care to arrive at a shared plan that all can support.

A case study is now provided to apply what we have been exploring. This study is realistic but represented by a hypothetical situation.

Case Study

Salvador Hernández is a 35-year-old male who immigrated to Canada 2 years ago from Columbia. He came with his wife, Anna, and their 10-year-old son, Juan. They have been living on social assistance and in subsidized housing in Toronto, Ontario, for the past year. Salvador is a very proud man and has been frustrated that he has been unable to gain employment and again be the breadwinner of his family. Salvador has also found gaining competence in English to be a difficult feat. In Columbia he was an engineer with a specialization in electrical engineering, but has been unable to gain recognition as an engineer in Canada. To do so would force him to return to university for up to 2 years. He gets depressed over the reality that he is likely to never realize his dream of returning to his profession, as he lacks the financial resources to undertake these studies.

Recently, his wife Anna informed him that she was pregnant. Although overjoyed by this new addition to his family, it also has added to his level of stress. He has also noticed recently that he is very thirsty a lot of the time and is going to the washroom frequently. This is a change in how his body normally behaves, so he is a bit worried as well. He has decided that these changes are just due to his current situation. He is also relieved that his previous insomnia has changed and he is wanting to sleep more and more, even during the day. Again he has decided this change in his sleeping pattern is just a 'catching up' and has dismissed it as a concern. He comes from a culture where men must be tough and not be emotional about such things.

After trying for over a year to find employment, he finally is offered an hourly-paying job in the construction industry as an electrician journeyman. However, his employer insists that he must have a physical examination to ensure his health state before starting work. Salvador thinks this is a waste of time, but he also wants the work, so he makes an appointment at the Primary Health Clinic near his home. This will be his first time seeking any health care in Canada.

Upon arriving at the clinic Salvador is greeted by a Spanish speaking receptionist. He is delighted and begins to feel a sense of comfort. He is then called by a person who introduces herself as Ellen, a nurse working in the clinic. She guides him into a private examination room and takes his blood pressure, temperature, and weight, and then leaves the room and says the doctor will be in soon. Salvador is left alone for about 10 minutes, during this time he begins to worry about whether the nurse found anything wrong with him. Her lack of sharing information about her findings makes him wonder and worry. In his country when people don't share information it usually means bad news. Finally, a male physician comes into his examination room who introduces himself as Dr. Walker. He asks Salvador what he has come for help with. Salvador explains in his broken English about his job and needing to have a checkup. Dr. Walker then asks Salvador about his health. Salvador reassures him that he is very healthy. Dr. Walker asks about whether he has ever had high blood pressure? Salvador becomes quite alarmed as to whether there is something wrong with him, and if this is what the nurse found when she was checking him.

Case Study Analysis

In the above scenario the fictitious case study demonstrates how some aspects of client health provider or staff member encounters can be very *supportive* and reassuring. The receptionist helped Salvador feel comfortable. However, when language is already a barrier and a client masks health issues of importance to only focus on the immediate need, in this case a clearance for work, in meeting with a physician, a more serious potential health issue might not be uncovered unless effective probing from the client occurs. Furthermore, when health providers do not create an environment of *openness* with clients and an in-depth understanding of their current situation, such as Ellen the nurse not sharing her assessment outcome, miscommunication and misunderstandings can occur; in this case, asking if Salvador was feeling anxious and mentioning that his blood pressure is a bit high may have led to the beginning of a meaningful dialogue between Salvador and the nurse. The quality of the nurse and physician interaction sets the atmosphere for discussion. In this case, the nurse could have explored with Salvador his narrative story providing a depth of understanding about his life situation to assist the nurse to explore and to integrate her findings about his blood pressure into their exchange. When only the task of taking the blood pressure occurs without such dialog, issues in his life that might be adding to his stress are lost. Furthermore, it appears to Salvador that (based on previous experiences) the nurse is withholding information from him, which further increased his anxiety and in turn increased his blood pressure. Hence, by the time the physician sees him and mentions his blood pressure, his symptoms are further elevated, which is likely to escalate his anxiety rather than reducing it. Thus demonstrating how a potentially therapeutic interaction may in fact escalate the symptoms.

The first encounter with a client by health providers sets the environment that the client believes they must fit into. An interaction between two parties can range from being a one-way exposition to a "two-way equal exchange of views" (Jarvis, 2012, p. 156). When health providers set the tone that they are the source of expertise to the client, there is a greater likelihood of limiting interactions to one-way exchanges. In Salvador's case, he is provided with the cues first by the nurse who simply takes monitoring parameters of his current condition without exploring with Salvador what life situations are associated with these parameters. Thus, a shared two-way exchange of views is never reached, which according to Jarvis (2012) is a requirement for learning. The one-way exchange of conversation continues when the physician comments on Salvador's blood pressure. As Jarvis suggested, this encounter creates in Salvador a "disjunctional experience" (2012, p. 156), in which Salvador tries to understand the meaning of this information, but may not have the language skills to ask about what this can mean for him, especially when he is starting a new job. The disjunctional experience is processed by Salvador using both internalization and externalization processes to create a meaning for him through the information provided by the physician (Le Cornu, 2009). However, if Salvador feels uncomfortable or unable to share how he is feeling about this information he may remain silent and just take any treatments or prescriptions for medication provided by the doctor. He may then return home and have to make a decision on whether he can or cannot afford any suggested treatments and further whether he believes that his elevated blood pressure is important for him to control.

In a real situation a full work up would have occurred since this was Salvador's first visit to the clinic and other health issues such as his increasing urination, fatigue, and thirst are likely to have been identified and acted upon. We have chosen to limit this depth for the purposes of understanding how patients, such as Salvador, might process a health encounter with health providers when faced with cultural and language limitations. These limitations are likely to further impact on his health literacy and ability to understand the meaning of interactive elements in a client–health provider scenario. For example, his cultural background may be attributed to males assuming the role of breadwinner and authority figure in the home. Such a role could influence him to avoid any discussion about what might be a perceived as a weakness in him.

Hence, in this scenario there is a beginning *engagement* with Salvador by the receptionist, the nurse, and the physician. The elements of engagement, according to Carman et al., (2013) include shared power and responsibility, clients acting as active partners in defining their goals and making decisions, bidirectional information flowing throughout the process, and sharing the decision-making responsibility. Florin, Ehrenberg, and Ehnfors (2008) suggest that when true engagement occurs an individualized tailoring of care results that is based on the client's readiness to be involved in his or her care. Readiness for care is associated with a willingness to change from a current state (that resulted in the health issues) to a state that incorporates modifications in the previous norm. Prochaska and Norcross (2001) developed and tested a typology for acceptance of change, including (from the lowest to highest level) (a) *precontemplation*, in which people do not know there is a need to change; (b) *contemplation*, in which people see current state is not healthy and considering making changes; (c) *preparation*, in which people make a plan to change; (d) *action*, in which people enact the plan; and (e) *maintenance*, in which the plan is enacted and continuing. In Salvador's case he is likely at a precontemplation stage, as when he came in for his appointment he did not even know he was experiencing high blood pressure. When a one-way exchange such as in our case scenario occurs, the likelihood of engagement characteristics existing may be absent. Hence, in this scenario, Salvador experienced the traditional health-provider-dominated interaction, which is not likely to lead to shared decision making or goal setting with Salvador by the end of this encounter. Engagement does provide the conditions for client participation in their care. However, often in the literature engagement is associated with clients who are experiencing chronic health challenges taking on their own self-care management and is not consistently attributed to an interactive sharing of ideas, experiences, and feelings about a client situation between health providers and clients. Two identified limitations to this level of engagement are time and resources.

Florin et al., (2008) developed an instrument to assist clients in understanding their preference for their role based on their control and comfort levels. The Control Preference Role Scale assesses the means for clients selecting their role within their health provider encounters as (a) *passive*, deferring to health providers for decisions; (b) *collaborating*, sharing in decision making with health providers; or (c) *active*, making decisions based on best evidence provided by health providers. These roles have some similarities to Hibbard et al.'s (2007) activation levels, but incorporate the relational aspects between clients and health providers. However, there is a paucity of work associated with what learning clients need to gain to collaborate and to become active partners with health providers in their care.

Health providers have traditionally practiced based on their professional knowledge and research evidence. Currently, pressures to improve health outcomes in populations are shifting health care to a more collaborative model between clients and health providers. Collaborative models require health providers to also shift in their role from sole professional to interprofessional team members that include clients' voices in their care. To refocus the engagement toward clients' participation in their care necessitates a change within health professionals' perspective on both the role of clients in their health care and health professionals' roles within interprofessional collaborative teams. To explore these shifts in relationships we must first focus on how care is currently provided and how it can become a collaborative practice.

CONCLUSION

In this chapter discussion has focused on the client and to some extent their family members within interprofessional collaborative practice. The reader has been provided with a number of different perspectives related to learning within these individuals and the influence of interactions between clients and health providers that has the potential to enhance their health. Limitations to enactment of this form of practice were discussed as well as a potential framework for this form of practice. Finally, the reader was provided with some insights into how to prepare clients and family members to their role as a member of interprofessional collaborative teams.

REFERENCES

Abma, T. A., & Broerse, J. E. W. (2010). Patient participation as dialogue: Setting research agendas. *Health Expectations, 13,* 160–173. http://dx.doi.org/10.1111/j.1369-7625.2009.00549.x.

Barello, S. Graffigna, G., & Vegni, E. (2012). Patient engagement as an emerging challenge for healthcare services: Mapping the literature. *Nursing Research & Practice, 2012,* 1–7. http://dx.doi.org/10.1155 /2012/905934.

Beach, M. C., & Inui, T. (2006). Perspectives: Relationship-centered care. A constructive reframing. *Journal of General Internal Medicine, 21*(Suppl. 1), S3–S8. http://dx.doi.org/10.1111/j.1525-1497.2006.00302.x.

Carman, K. L., Dardess, P., Maurer, M., Sofaer, S., Adams, K., Bechtel, C., & Sweeney, J. (2013). Patient and family engagement: A framework for understanding the elements and developing interventions and policies. *Health Affairs, 32,* 223-231. http://dx.doi.org/10.1377/hlthaff.2012.1133.

Clancy, C. M. (2011). Patient engagement in health care. *Health Services Research, 46*(2), 389–393. http://dx.doi.org/10.1111/j.1475-6773.2011.01254.x.

Coulter, A. (1999). Paternalism or partnership? Patients have grown up: And there's no going back. *British Medical Journal, 319*, 719-720. http://dx.doi.org/10.1136/bmj.319.7212.719.

Coulter, A. (2012). Patient engagement – What works? *Journal of Ambulatory Care Management, 35*(2), 80–89. http://dx.doi.org/10.1097/ JAC.0b013e318249e0fd.

Florin, J., Ehrenberg, A., & Ehnfors, M. (2008). Clinical decision-making: Predictors of patient participation in nursing care. *Journal of Clinical Nursing, 17*, 2935–2944. http://dx.doi.org/10.1111/j.1365-2702.2008.02328.x.

Frank, C., Asp, M., & Dahlberg, K. (2008). Patient participation in emergency care – a phenomenographic analysis of caregivers' conceptions. *Journal of Clinical Nursing, 18*, 2555–2562. http://dx.doi.org/10.1111/j.1365-2702.2008.02477.x.

Gittell, J. H., Godfrey, M., & Thistlethwaite, J. (2013). Interprofessional collaborative practice and relational coordination: Improving healthcare through relationships. *Journal of Interprofessional Care, 27*, 210–213. http://dx.doi.org/10.3109/13561820.2012.730564.

Gruman, J., Rovner, M. H., French, M. E., Jeffress, D. Sofaer, S., Shaller, D., & Prager, D. J. (2010). From patient education to patient engagement: Implications for the field of patient education. *Patient Education and Counseling, 78,* 350–356. http://dx.doi.org/10.1016/j.pec.2010.02.002.

Haigh, C. A. (2008). Exploring the evidence base of patient involvement in the management of health care services. *Journal of Nursing Management, 16*, 452–462. http://dx.doi.org/10.1111/j.1365-2834.2008.00865.x.

Henderson, S. (2003). Power imbalance between nurses and patients: A potential inhibitor of partnerships in care. *Journal of Clinical Nursing, 12*, 501–508. Http://dx.doi.org/10.1046/j.1365-2702.2003.00757.x.

Hibbard, J. H., Mahoney, E. R., Stock, R., & Tusler, M. (2007). Do increases in patient activation result in improved self-management behaviors? *Health Services Research, 42*, 1443–1463. http://dx.doi.org/10.1111/ j.1475-6773.2006.00669.x.

Jarvis, P. (2012). *Learning to be a person in society.* London, United Kingdom: Routledge.

Le Cornu, A. (2009). Meaning, internalization, and externalization: Toward a fuller understanding of the process of reflection and its role in the construction of the self. *Adult Education Quarterly, 59*, 279–297. http://dx.doi.org/10.1177/0741713609331478.

Lee, S.-Y. D., Arozullah, A. M., & Cho, Y. I. (2004). Health literacy, social support, and health: A research agenda. *Social Science & Medicine, 58*, 1309–1321. http://dx.doi.org/10.1016/S0277-9536(03)00329-0.

Longtin, Y., Sax, H., Leape, L. L, Sheridan, S. E., Donaldson, L., & Pittet, D. (2010). Patient participation: Current knowledge and applicability of patient safety. *Mayo Clinical Procedures, 85*, 53–62. http://dx.doi.org/10.4065/mcp.2009.0248.

Martin, G. P. (2011). The third sector, user involvement and public service reform: A case study in the co-governance of health service provision. *Public Administration, 89*, 909–932. http://dx.doi.org/10.1111/j.1467-9299.2011.01910.x.

Moss-Morris, R., Weinman, K., Petrie, L. K., Horne, R., Cameron, L. D., & Buick, D. (2002). The revised illness perception questionnaire (IOPQ-R). *Psychology and Health, 17*, 1–16.

Prochaska, J. O., & Norcross, J. C. (2001). Stages of change. *Psychotherapy, 38,* 443–448. http://dx.doi.org/10.1037/0033-3204.38.4.443.

Riegel, B., Jaarsma, T., & Strömberg, A. (2012). Middle-range theory of self-care of chronic illness. *Advances in Nursing Science, 35*(3), 194–204. http://dx.doi.org/10.1097/ANS.0b013e318261b1ba

Sahlsten, M. J. M., Larsson, I. E., Sjöström, B., & Plos, K. A. (2008). An analysis of the concept of patient participation. *Nursing Forum, 43*(1), 2–11. http://dx.doi.org/10.1111/j.1744-6198.2008.00090.x.

Sahlsten, M. J. M., Larsson, I. E., Sjöström, B., & Plos, K. A. (2009). Nurse strategies for optimizing patient participation in nursing care. *Scandinavian Journal of Clinical Science, 23,* 490–497. http://dx.doi.org/10.1111/j.1471-6712.2008.00649.x

Saunders, P. (1995). Encouraging patients to take part in their own care. *Nursing Times, 91*(9), 42–43.

Tomson, R., Murtagh, M., & Khaw, F.-M. (2005). Tensions in public health policy: Patient engagement, evidence-based public health and health inequalities. *Quality Safety Health Care, 14,* 398–400. http://dx.doi.org/10.1136/qshc.2005.014175

University of Western Ontario, Office of the Interprofessional Health Education & Research. (2015). *Patient/client.* Retrieved from http://www.ipe.uwo.ca/Professionals/patient.html

World Health Organization. (2014). Global status report on noncommunicable diseases 2014. Geneva: Author. http://www.who.int/nmh/publications/ncd-status-report-2014/en/

In: Interprofessional Client-Centred Collaborative Practice   ISBN: 978-1-63483-754-5
Editor: Carole Orchard   © 2015 Nova Science Publishers, Inc.

Chapter 2

WHAT IS COMPETENCE IN CLIENT-CENTERED COLLABORATIVE PRACTICE?

Carole Orchard[1] and Lesley Bainbridge[2]
[1]Western University, London, ON, Canada
[2]University of British Columbia, Vancouver, BC, Canada

ABSTRACT

This chapter provides an overview of the topic of competence in general usage and then in professional practice and its application into interprofessional client-centered collaborative practice. Collaboration is then discussed as both an outcome and a process. This follows a discussion related to the four approaches that can be adopted to assess competence. The reader is then presented with an in depth discussion of the CIHC Interprofessional Collaboration Competency Framework and of its competency domains and descriptors. A case study is provided within the chapter to present how each of the competencies may be demonstrated within a primary health care team environment.

Keywords: Competence, competencies, capability, core competencies, domain competence, subject competence, personal competence, social competence

INTRODUCTION

Over the past two decades authors have presented arguments and counterarguments on how to define competence. Competence is viewed in a variety of ways as (a) an area of work (Moore, Cheng, & Dainty, 2002); (b) developmental and elaborative (Hackett, 2001); (c) associated with personal traits, tasks people do, or outcomes needed for work (Mansfield, 2004); (d) comprising technical, professional, managerial, human, and conceptual aspects (Derouen & Kleiner, 1994); and (e) as worker oriented, work oriented, or multidimensional (Grzeda, 2005). To be competent requires meeting a standard of practice, which reflects an adequate level of skill to enact a role.

The level to which an individual can demonstrate competence is not the same concept as the competencies that define individual characteristics, characteristics of an organization, or tools to set conditions to assist educators in preparing those for the labor market (Garavan & McGuire, 2001). Competencies are often presented in a variety of classifications, including core competencies associated with an organization's ability to deliver its services, functional competencies that link job roles to their enactment in organizations, or specific competencies identifying what an individual is expected to bring into the workplace to perform effectively (Le Deist & Winterton, 2005). Professions also often use the terms core or essential competencies to describe professional standards of practice. In education settings, most graduates of health professional programs are expected to demonstrate proficiency in specific competencies in order to enter into their professional practice roles. In practice settings, employers provide job descriptions that specify functional competencies for employees to enact within the organization.

Hence, there is a myriad of ways that the terms competence and competencies are used. Le Deist and Winterton (2005) suggest dividing competencies into those associated with functional and those associated with behavioral areas of performance. However, Stoof, Martens, van Merriënboer, and Bastiaens (2002) see this as too simplistic and present a counterargument by suggesting a framework to guide how one views competence and competencies, which they term the "boundary approach" (p. 345). In this framework, Stoof et al., suggest that when you view competence that combines its demonstration in the task provided and a person's own knowledge and understanding associated with the task, then a definition of competence is related to an individual's own competence that he or she brings into practice, which is termed "inside-out" (p. 354). An example of inside-out competence is when an employer considers a person to be hired for a position. In contrast, when the focus is on how well a person performs tasks and evidence of the person's knowledge, skills, attributes, and abilities are part of this, the focus on competence is deemed to be from the "outside-in" (Stoof et al., 2002, p. 358). An example of outside-in competence is when a supervisor assesses a staff member's performance. Cheetham and Chivers (1996) proposed an earlier "holistic model of professional competence" (p. 24) comprising cognitive competence (to know and understand), functional competence (skills to be demonstrated), personal competence (knowing behavioral expectations), ethical competence (applying values), and meta-competence (coping with situations). Le Deist and Winterton (2005) support the above debate and suggest the need to view competence through a meta-competence lens that contains additive components of cognitive, functional, and social competence.

Setting aside the nomenclature arguments about how to classify competence, we return to how professional competence (often in the form of sets of competencies) is commonly described. The most common components are associated with the knowledge, skills, attitudes, and values that an individual brings to his or her practice from both professional standards of practice and from personal social learning. Hence, competencies, as Travis (2002) suggests,

> provide (i) quality standards for professional workplace training and development, (ii) benchmarks for assessing the competence of ... professionals, (iii) a framework for evidence-based practice, (iv) benchmarks for measuring service quality and (v) "real world" learning outcomes and assessment criteria for professional education programs. (p. 269)

Other authors suggest that the use of competencies is too limiting to reflect the complexity and uncertainty in today's practice, which often requires rapid and time-sensitive decisions and actions. These authors suggest the use of capabilities rather than competencies to support practice performance. Capability has been defined "as an integrated application of knowledge where the student or practitioner can adapt to change, develop new behaviours and continue to improve performance" (Walsh, Gordon, Marshall, Wilson, & Hunt, 2005, p. 28) and further as "the extent to which individuals can apply, adapt and synthesize new knowledge in different service contexts" (Fraser & Greenhalgh, 2001, p. 799). Physician practice development currently reflects "entrustable professional activities" (ten Cate & Scheele, 2007, p. 79-80, which seems to also reflect a capability approach. Others have suggested that capabilities of individuals to practice is a more valuable approach, while still others supporting this position suggest the competencies are only associated with less-than-expert level of practice. Garavan and McGuire (2001) as well as Stoof et al., (2002) settle this debate by stating capability is but a component of competence, albeit an important one.

To date, a growing number of core competency frameworks have been developed, approved by various regulators and professions, and applied to performance of members. These frameworks apply to professional standards as well as to context-specific competencies that cross professional boundaries such as patient safety and public health. More recently, the Canadian Interprofessional Health Collaborative (2010) released its *Interprofessional Collaboration Competency Framework,* and the American Interprofessional Education Collaborative (2011) released its *Core Competencies for Interprofessional Collaborative Practice*. These latter two frameworks align with professional entry to practice competencies. Hence, the use of competencies to define performance standards has become a common approach to performance measurement far beyond just education and health care. In this chapter, we will discuss how competencies and competence are perceived by team members within a professional perspective, how trust is developed within teams, and finally we will explore some examples of interprofessional competency or capability frameworks. These discussions will be embedded within a case example.

CASE STUDY

Samira Jarvis is a 29-year-old family practice first-year resident who has been placed in the Golden River Family Health Team. Samira is excited to have this opportunity since the team is composed of 2 Family Physicians, 2 Nurse Practitioners, 1 Registered Nurse, 1 Dietitian, 1 Social Worker, the clinical administrator, and a receptionist. While in her medical school undergraduate program, Samira was well oriented to the CanMEDs competencies for physicians. She also participated in some interprofessional workshops, in which she learned about the roles of these other health professionals. However, she has some concerns about how these other team members will accept her into their environment. Samira asked the Family Medicine Post-Graduate Placement Coordinator how to prepare to fit into this group. The Coordinator seemed surprised by her question and suggested she talk to the Clinic Administrator and provided her with contact information. The administrator indicated that Samira would be oriented to the work when she arrived. On the morning of her first day in the clinic she was met by one of the Family Physicians who introduced her to a set of guidelines that the total team had created. He indicated that the team operates as a collaborative group and reflects on their teamwork using the Canadian Interprofessional Health Collaborative's (CIHC) Interprofessional Competency Framework and asked if Samira was familiar with this. She indicated yes she had learned about the CIHC competencies in a couple of workshops she attended at the university where she did her undergraduate medical education. Samira felt a sense of excitement to be working with a collaborative team and looked forward to this placement as an excellent learning experience for herself.

As a new team member Samira might anticipate that she will need to earn trust from the other team members, and in turn she will need to learn to trust them. Trust will develop in response to how Samira presents her competence to the other team members. Her quest to become a valued member of the team begins with her gaining an understanding of the guidelines that the team has for working with each other.

Golden River Family Health Team Guidelines for Teamwork
As a collaborative team we strive to --

- Provide excellence in patient-centered care.
- Support collaboration and partnerships with ourselves and with our patients and their families.
- Ensure we are consistently respectful to each other and those who come for our care and services.
- Accept shared accountability for the care or services we provide.
- Encourage each other and our patients and their families to find innovative solutions to health and social challenges.
- Work towards care and services that are continuously reviewed to enhance their quality.

Samira is pleased to see the guidelines that the team uses to inform the way they practice. She also considers how these will apply to the collaborator role in the CanMed's competencies (Frank, Snell, & Sherbino, 2015). The competency states, "Physicians work effectively with other health care professionals to provide safe, high-quality, patient-centred care" (p. 7). To enable competencies,

Physicians are able to:

- Establish and maintain positive relationships with physicians and other colleagues in the health care professions to support relationship-centred collaborative care
- Negotiate overlapping and shared responsibilities with physicians and other colleagues in the health care professions in episodic and ongoing care
- Engage in respectful shared decision-making with physicians and other colleagues in the health care professions. (Frank et al., 2015, p. 8)

Samira realizes that there is consistency between the Golden River Family Health Team (GRFHT) guidelines for teamwork and her own physician competencies, which will assist her when her performance is evaluated by her preceptor and other members of the team. Samara's challenge is to ensure that she is able to demonstrate her competence in her family physician role. Competence is "the habitual and judicious use of communication, knowledge, technical skills, clinical reasoning, emotions, values, individual and community being served" (Epstein

& Hundert, 2002, p. 226). Samira realizes that she will need to demonstrate two types of competencies within the team — foundational and functional. Her foundational competencies are related to her knowledge, skills, attitudes, and values, while her functional competencies relate to how she will perform in her role. As a new team member she will be assessed on what she brings to her work (input), what she does in her role (process), and what she is able to achieve (output) (Greenhalgh & Macfarlane, 1997).

> **COMPETENCE IN PRACTICE is associated with:**
>
> **INPUT** – What a team member brings to practice
>
> **PROCESS** – What a team member does in his or her role
>
> **OUTPUT** – What a team member is able to achieve

A person's competence is influenced by time, experience, and the context of practice (Frank et al., 2010). Samira also realizes that she must demonstrate her integrity as a physician in order to earn the trust of team members. Hence her capacity to demonstrate her practice integrity is dependent on her level of expertise, her responsibility for care decision making, and the domain of practice within which she is practicing (Khomeiran, Yekta, Kiger, & Ahmadi, 2006). The ability to demonstrate competence is associated with three components of competence — domain or subject, personal, and social competence.

Domain or Subject Competence

Domain or subject competence is associated with Samara's willingness or ability to carry out tasks and solve problems as a physician (Le Deist & Winterton, 2005). These tasks are also reflected in entrustable professional activities. Researchers ten Cate and Schelle (2007) identified a set of conditions that support the development and enactment of entrustable professional activities, which include the following:

1. Is part of essential professional work in a given context.
2. Must require adequate knowledge, skill, and attitude.
3. Must lead to recognized output of professional labor.
4. Should be confined to qualified personnel.
5. Should be independently executable.
6. Should be executable within a time frame.
7. Should be observable and measurable in its process and outcome ... .
8. Should reflect one or more competencies (p. 545).

Samara realizes that she needs to consider her entrustable professional activities within the context of interprofessional collaborative teamwork. Hence, she will need to learn the skills, knowledge, and expertise of other team members and determine how she will need to negotiate and adapt to the shared work of the team.

Walsh et al., (2005) extended subject competence to interprofessional teamwork and suggested, "Teamwork includes awareness of others' professional regulations, structures, functions and processes of the team within an environment of anti-discriminatory non-judgmental practice" (p. 235). According to Salas, DiazGranados, Weaver, and King (2008), effective collaboration requires that interprofessional team members be provided with team-building opportunities outside their normal patient care work. These opportunities require team members to practice their interprofessional skills and to receive feedback from each other on the effectiveness of their skill demonstration.

When a group of health professionals comes together to focus on the care needs of individual patients there is a shared set of competencies required in relation to their interprofessional communications, patient assessment, client care planning, monitoring of care implementation, and advocacy on behalf of the client and each other (Reeves, Fox, & Hodges, 2009). Interprofessional communication seems to emerge consistently as a critical element in effective interprofessional teamwork. However, the question remains, what constitutes effective interprofessional communications? In a study of nurse-physician communications in a hospital setting, Robinson, Gorman, Slimmer, and Yudkowsky (2010) found that clarity and precision in messaging was dependent on how well team members verified and confirmed the messages they receive. It is also dependent on how well the team members collaboratively problem solve in a client situation and on members' abilities to maintain mutual respect and a calm demeanor no matter how stressful the situation may be. It is also critical that all team members understand and value each other's role. Conn et al., (2009) identified both synchronous and asynchronous communications that occur as scheduled and unscheduled interactions between team members. They found that synchronous interprofessional communications were mostly unplanned and led to more in-depth planning around client care (Conn et al., 2009). The scheduled events occurred often through charting or client rounds, while the unscheduled events occurred through impromptu hallway discussions (Conn et al., 2009). Health professionals seem to depend on their organization's formal communication systems to meet their needs. When these are inadequate, they tend to rely on unplanned opportunistic situations to discuss client care that may never transfer into the formal systems. Interprofessional teamwork needs to focus on the communication structures that all interprofessional team members will use to ensure effective communications occur. Thus, part of team building needs to address the timing, the means, the content, and the distribution of communications across a team. This can be accomplished through the use of communication guidelines.

Samira explored with some of the team members how they manage to effectively communicate with each other. One of the nurses explained that initially there was a lot of miscommunication among team members. As a group, they explored how to create a consistent way to communicate. This resulted in the group adopting the situation, background, assessment, and recommendation (SBAR) template. Samira had heard people talk about SBAR before, but was not sure how it helped with communications. The nurse explained that she too was unfamiliar with it until she attended an interprofessional workshop where it was used. She explained that the *S* was about a brief description of the situation, the *B* is a brief overview about the background to the client situation you are seeking help with, the *A* is your own assessment of the situation, and the *R* are your recommendations. She further explained how this approach has enhanced communication and the comprehensiveness of information that is shared by and with each team member. The nurse then directed Samira to a number of websites related to the SBAR approach to information sharing. Samara decided that she would explore its adoption and start trying to use it herself in the team. However, this serendipitous conversation with her nursing colleague had alerted Samira to the use of the SBAR approach, not a formal orientation to it. Without the conversation she would likely have continued to communicate in the way she had previously learned. This may have put Samira in a difficult position with the team who may have judged her for her lack of knowledge about SBAR, when in fact the problem resides with the team and the orientation provided to new members. If agreed-upon principles and approaches are not shared with and followed by mentoring new members, collaborative teamwork will fail.

Personal Competence

Personal competence reflects the willingness and ability of individuals to understand, analyze, and judge their day-to-day lives and plans. To be personally competent requires that people have a level of comfort in their independence of thinking and are able to critically judge their own behavior and skills. They have a level of self-confidence and demonstrate reliability as well as the ability to be responsible for what they agree to do within their scope of practice.

Social Competence

Social competence reflects a willingness and ability to enter into and shape relationships with others. Social competence requires personal competence as well as subject competence. In interprofessional collaborative teams social competence is enacted through teamwork. McNair (2005) stated that health professional education poorly prepares students for their teamwork roles; however, significant efforts have been made since 2005 to provide understanding about the various roles in health care. Several researchers have carried out studies to identify the key competencies for interprofessional collaborative practice, including communication, strength in one's professional role, knowledge of professional role of others, leadership, team function, and negotiation for conflict resolution (Macdonald et al., 2010), and understanding and appreciating professional roles and responsibilities, and communicating effectively (Suter et al., 2009).

Team Practice Environment and Individual Fit

The ability to develop competence in collaboration is associated with several factors:

- Experience – the more experience one has the greater the competence,
- Opportunities – opportunities that challenge abilities and performance enhance competence,

- Environment – competence is more likely to evolve when mutual respect, partnership, support and trust is shown to each other,
- Personal characteristics – competence is enhanced when current practices are questioned and when mentoring is provided to each other,
- Motivation – competence is enhanced when an individual is motivated to demonstrate the means to improve another's outcomes,
- Theoretical knowledge – competence is enhanced when an individual seeks out new learning associated with practice questions (Khomeiran et al., 2006, pp. 68–69).

Fitting into the team is associated with a match between individuals' values, what is important to them about their practice, their underlying belief systems, and their views related to how practice should be carried out. When team members' perspectives related to the above are shared among the team of health professionals they become the team's norms of practice (Arford & Zone-Smith, 2005).

Cognitive-based trust in teamwork is, according to Lee (2004), a "rational evaluation of an individual's ability to carry out obligations ... [and] reflects beliefs about that individual's reliability, dependability, and competency" (p. 625). Affective-based trust is that which "reflects an emotional attachment that stems from care and concern that exist between individuals" (Lee, 2004, p. 625). Hence, trusting another team member requires a willingness to take risks by cooperating with that individual and a willingness to refrain from controlling and monitoring other team members (Costa, 2003). When strong cognitive trust is present in teams, there is a reduction in errors within the team (Erdem & Ozen, 2003). Development of trust within collaborative teams has been associated with perceptions of members' competence in their professional and interprofessional practice. Cooperative behaviors and perceived trustworthiness have been shown to be strong elements of effective teamwork (Costa, 2003). Erdem and Ozen (2003) found that when team members begin working together or when there is a change in members within the team, team members focus on the new members' competence by assessing their integrity and ability to fit into the team's norms of practice. Once team members' competence is accepted, then affective-based trust is enacted as relationships develop.

Nevertheless, other authors have suggested that focusing on specific types of competence is limiting. Health care providers need to consider approaches that are inclusive of all types of competence resulting in meta-competence.

Approaches to Competency Frameworks

Over time, four different approaches may be used when exploring competency frameworks: skill based, life-skills based, competency based, and integrative. Each of these is explored in the following subsections.

Skill-based competency frameworks group together several specific objectives for practice, then determine the skills required to meet the objectives, and the assessment of outcome focuses on meeting the objectives. Supporters of this approach suggest that the practice allows for a set of common core competencies that are reflective of the individual's scope and requirements for practice. They further allow for delineation of the various roles and what the performance expectations of individuals holding this role are expected to demonstrate.

Life-skills based frameworks focus on how people develop their capacity to actively exercise their role as a member of a society. For example, this may include how a client is expected to behave within health care teams and how a professional gains personal experiences that further shape how the individual enacts his or her professional role. Thus, within a life-skills perspective knowing is gained through experiential learning that is often guided by societal values and expectations. Hence, professionals bring both their professional skill-based learning and their experiential learning into their practice, and this shapes how they each view a client encounter and contribute to formulating a shared plan of care.

Competency-based frameworks are shaped by the knowledge and skills individuals have gained and how their enactment results in outcomes. Competence using this approach focuses only on outcomes and not on the process that supported the achievement of the outcome. Hence, competency-based frameworks are associated with the 'knowledge to act' achieved as an outcome. Interventions are the drivers that help to achieve the outcomes. One other feature of competency-based frameworks is that they allow for each outcome achieved to be assessed. Therefore, the importance is not the learning in itself, but how the learning helped achievement of the outcome.

An integrative approach uses a framework that values all of the above three types of competency frameworks. It incorporates skills, life-skills, and competency-based approaches through integrating knowledge, skills, attitudes, and values in order to make judgments about future actions. Roegiers (2007) is one of the proponents of this approach and advocates for learners to focus on situations they encounter in which they are either invited or required to respond using their knowledge and life skills as the resources they need to assess, interpret, and respond to the situation. Thus, the integrative approach recognizes the capacity of individuals to respond in situations of complexity and uncertainly using the knowledge, skills, values, and previous experiences to provide a means to address the situation in a given context.

APPLICATION OF AN INTEGRATIVE PEDAGOGICAL APPROACH TO INTERPROFESSIONAL COLLABORATIVE PRACTICE

The CIHC's (2010) Interprofessional Competency Working Group incorporated Roegier's (2007) integrative pedagogy into its national framework. The challenge during the framework development phase was in finding an approach that would allow collaboration within teams to be demonstrated through identified competencies. Since collaboration can be viewed as both an outcome and a process, CIHC decided that other interprofessional competencies already focused on outcomes, but the need to understand the process teams undertake to enact collaborative practice seemed to be of higher importance. The integrative pedagogical approach takes into account team members' shared knowledge, skills, attitudes, and values in order to arrive at the best team judgment related to care for their clients based on their shared contributions. The development of team judgments are also shaped by characteristics of the nature of competence identified by Tardif (1999): it is complex (dynamic organization of competencies); additive (integration of knowledge, skills, attitudes, and values to formulate judgments); integrative (dependent on the shared contributions of the team members); developmental (moves from novice to expert over time); and evolutionary (applied within a given context leading to ongoing new understandings). Thus, both Roegier's integrative pedagogy along with Tardif's characteristics provide a means to address how a comprehensive framework for assessment of competencies can evolve.

In the CIHC (2010) *Interprofessional Competency Framework*, the competencies evolve from and are foundational to the central goal, which is interprofessional collaborative practice. There are six competencies: (a) client/family/community-centered care, in which "practitioners seek out, integrate and value, as a partner, the input, and the engagement of the patient/client/family, community in designing and implementing care/services" (p. 13); (b) interprofessional communication, in which "practitioners from different professions communicate with each other in a collaborative, responsive, and responsible manner" (p. 16); (c) role clarification, in which "practitioners understand their own role and the roles of those in others professions, and use this knowledge appropriately to establish and achieve patient/client/family and community goals" (p. 12); (d) team functioning, in which "practitioners understand the principles of team work dynamics and group/team processes to enable effective interprofessional collaboration" (p. 14); (e) interprofessional conflict resolution, in which "practitioners actively engage self and others, including the client/patient/family, in positively and constructively addressing disagreements as they arise" (p. 17); and (f) collaborative leadership, in which "practitioners understand and can apply leadership principles that support a collaborative practice model" (p. 15).

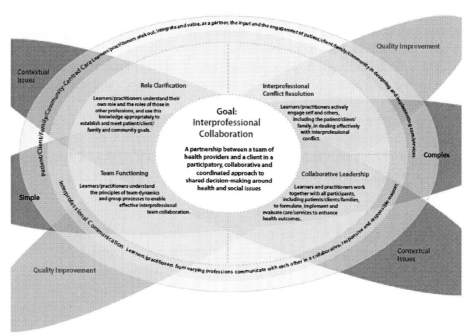

Note. From *A National Interprofessional Competency Framework* (p. 11), by the Canadian Interprofessional Health Collaborative, 2010, Vancouver, Canada: Author. Copyright 2010 by the Canadian Interprofessional Health Collaborative. Reprinted with permission.

Figure I. The Canadian Interprofessional Health Collaborative's (2010) Interprofessional Collaboration Competency Framework.

The CIHC (2010) framework's central goal of *interprofessional collaboration* is further described as "a partnership between a team of health professionals and a client in a participatory, collaborative and coordinated approach to shared decision-making around health and social issues" (Orchard, Curran, & Kabene, 2005, p. 1) and provides the processes needed for achievement of this goal. The focus of interprofessional collaborative practice is on providing client-centered care, which requires demonstration of interprofessional communication between and across health professionals with clients and families, necessitating an understanding of each other's roles inclusive of each person's knowledge, skills, and expertise that represents shared teamwork, an understanding of how team functioning is achieved through adoption of collaborative (shared) leadership, and team members' abilities to address and resolve interprofessional conflicts (see Figure I. Each of these competencies will be discussed below.

Patient/Client/Family/Community-Centered Care

In patient/client/family-centered care the client initiates care by bringing a health problem to health providers when the client's own resources are not felt to address the issue effectively. Interactions with health providers then integrate the expertise that the client brings with health providers' expertise in order to address the issue and to reduce the impact it is having on the client's functioning and quality of life. In this scenario the client is the driver for his or her health care, and the health providers are the mediators of the resources and expertise available to assist the client to address the health problem. A shared understanding of both parties' perspectives is required in order to reshape potential treatment options into choices that the client and his or her family members or chosen caregivers are able to manage. The combination of the client setting the agenda for his or her health issues and the health provider's need to fit evidence-informed practice into the client's and his or her family's realities is key to client-centered care. The only way in which such shared approaches can be achieved is when the client, his or her family members, or chosen care givers are invited in as integral members of the care team and are not viewed as outside responders to the health provider's suggested interventions. Patient/client/family-centered care is

> a partnership between a team of health providers and a client where the client retains control over his/her care and is provided access to the knowledge and skills of team members to arrive at a realistic team shared plan of care and access to the resources to achieve the plan (Orchard, 2009).

There is some emerging evidence that when clients, especially those with chronic health diseases, are provided with active participation in their care, they report high levels of satisfaction and feelings of empowerment (Adams, Orchard, Houghton, & Ogrin, 2014) and embrace higher levels of self-care management of their health (Hibbard, Mahoney, Stock, & Tusler, 2007).

Samara remembered how important it is in collaborative practice to authentically include the client as part of the team. She notes a new client, Philip Jordan, is scheduled for a one-hour intake appointment. Samara asks the receptionist, Jane, about what she has learned so far about Philip. Jane comments that he is a diabetic who is currently having trouble with his glycemic control. He recently moved to Golden River and needs to find a new physician. Samara realizes that Philip could benefit from a team meeting with her, as well as with Shawn who previously worked as a nurse diabetes educator and Philomena the clinic dietitian who could be very helpful in creating a plan for working with Philip. Samara sends a quick text message to Shawn and Philomena to see if they would be available to meet with her and Philip when he comes for his appointment later in the day. They quickly respond back that they can move things to be available. Samara is very pleased, as she believes that this approach will provide a higher quality of care plan to assist Philip. Samara wonders how often such team meetings occur in the clinic. She enters a note on her tablet to check this out later.

Achievement of the above competency by health providers can be a challenge to their existing approaches to client involvement in their health care. It also is a challenge to the role of the client. Samara reminds herself that she will need to ask Philip if he will be comfortable with both Shawn and Philomena attending his care discussions. Overall, Samara realizes how important using effective communication between health team members and their clients and families is to interprofessional client-centered collaborative practice.

Interprofessional Communication

Team communications are composed of shared information among health providers as well as among clients, their family, or chosen caregivers and health care providers. Communications comprise two components: content and relationships. Content relates to what is discussed, while relationships focus on how the senders and receivers feel about each other. These relationships are associated with four factors: (a) *affinity* — connection to one another; (b) *immediacy* — interest or attention to what is being said; (c) *respect* — degree of respect shared between the parties; and (d) *control* — amount of control one party exerts over another during interactions. The patterns for communicating within teams by health providers arise from their professional socialization (i.e., language, sharing information, and approaches to care) and are both unique to each profession and may be shared across other professions (Adler & Proctor, 2010). When communication patterns are not understood by another provider it can lead to patient safety issues (Baker et al., 2004; Institute of Medicine [IOM], 2001) and errors in care decision making (Robinson et al., 2010).

Interprofessional communication is only as effective as the quality of the information being shared and the shared understandings that exist between and among the team members involved in the interactions. Robinson et al., (2010) found that effective communication is reported when (a) clarity and precision is provided and when the parties verify the intent of the information; (b) collaborative problem solving between the parties occurs; (c) delivery of the information is carried out calmly and supportively between the parties particularly in stressful situations; and (d) when mutual respect exists between the parties from an authentic understanding of each other's role.

Samara considered the GRFHT's use of SBAR for their communications and realized how valuable having this consistent approach was to ensuring all the members could understand what was being shared. She realized also that just receiving an SBAR message was insufficient to ensure clarity of the information contained. She learned the importance of contacting the sender and exploring each of the components to ensure she had a shared understanding of the messaging. Samara also wondered how she could extend the use of SBAR into her team approach to inclusion of the patient and family in shaping care. She realized she needed to explore this more at the next team meeting.

Competence in interprofessional communication is essential for effective interactions with health providers and for ensuring that quality care is provided within a context of safety and their patient abilities. Hence, each member of the team will exercise a role within the team to assist in ensuring care is provided within a context of safe practices and at the highest quality possible within existing resources.

Role Clarification

Role understanding within interprofessional teams is key to supporting the development of trusting relationships. The focus to date has been on health providers' roles, but there is emerging attention to the role of the client and his or her family members or chosen caregivers within the team. The role of the client within the team is to "expresses her/his lived experience of illness or injury ... and its impact on his/her daily life and how suggested treatments and/or actions can be adapted (or not) into their activities of daily living" (University of Western Ontario, Office of the Interprofessional Health Education & Research, 2014, "What Can the Patient," para. 1). The family member or caregiver plays a complementary role to the client and "brings his/her understanding of [the patient's/client's] health and social needs and ensures these are recognized within ... [the patient's/client's] own frame of reference in the interaction [when necessary] with health and social care providers to assist in shaping a plan to address, monitor and reduce/resolve the identified issues" (University of Western Ontario, Office of the Interprofessional Health Education & Research, 2014, "Education," para. 1).

Team members need to gain a clear understanding of the knowledge, skills, and expertise that other health providers in the team can bring to their shared work. Such sharing often results in the ability for team members to use each other's shared areas of knowledge, skills, and expertise to assist in balancing workloads when required. In collaborative interprofessional teamwork, role clarification is an ongoing process (Adams et al., 2014). Roles gained by virtue of regulated practice are but one aspect; while these roles are considered a health provider's unique role predicated on specific training and competence, there are clearly areas of shared practice. The team must effectively match roles and needs and negotiate shared roles to best meet the needs of the client and team. The unique role is termed a focal role, and it is how a health provider takes professional knowledge, skills, and values and adapts them to the needs of the client being cared for within a team perspective (Orchard & Rykhoff, 2015).

The need for team members to share their knowledge and skills from each of their perspectives and then arrive at an agreed, shared approach is an example of how role clarification results in an actual client care situation. Enactment of role clarification in which all members value, respect, and support each other's agreed-upon responsibilities in a care situation is essential in order for trust to develop in teams. Role clarification provides a critical means for team members to function as a collaborative group.

Team Functioning

Interprofessional collaborative teams can be found in any health care setting and are composed of any number of members from small to large. Members' duration in the team and relationships with colleagues in the team enhance the capacity for collaborative teamwork. Components associated with team functioning include team context and structure (i.e., working environment and team coordinating mechanisms), team processes (i.e., the means that team members adopt to support collaborative work), and team outcomes or how well set goals were achieved (Deneckere et al., 2011). The effectiveness of collaborative teams is associated with members' participation and commitment to the team, team objectives, team's clarity and orientation to their tasks, and team members' support for innovation (West & Field, 1995.) Team effectiveness necessitates its members learning to work interdependently in support of shared goals through collaborative discussions and decision making about both their teamwork and their shared treatment approaches with their clients.

The maturing of a collaborative team evolves through what Howarth, Warner, and Haigh (2012) call member reciprocal *respect* and *trust*. Respect and trust among the members allows for the evolution of a *collective efficacy* to their work; this in turn supports client-centered goal sharing among the team members, which results in a *conditional partnership* within the team membership. Conditional partnerships, according to Howarth et al., lead to a *perceived team credibility* by each member. Continuance of team credibility is predicated on members feeling that their input is valued, sought out, and used within the team, resulting in each member continuing to contribute to the team efforts. If their perceived value decreases, their conditional partnership may end and team members may distance themselves from the team (Howarth et al., 2012).

Creating team structures, processes, and outcomes necessitates team members taking time out of their client care practice to develop teamwork skills through group training (Adams et al., 2014; Salas et al., 2008). Ongoing work to maintain their agreed-upon team functioning is essential for members to maintain and strengthen team credibility. Furthermore, attention to orientation of new members into the team is critical to the ongoing effectiveness of collaborative teamwork. Achieving effective team functioning necessitates members addressing how to develop shared leadership and support from their formal manager (Orchard & Rykhoff, 2015).

Samara realized when her colleagues agreed to work with her on Philip's care that her colleagues welcome interprofessional team functioning. She decides to approach those structures, processes, and outcomes that the team had agreed to in a forthcoming team meeting to gain better insight into the team's functioning to ensure she fits into their practice.

Collaborative and Shared Leadership

The capacity of a collaborative team to share in team leadership is an outcome of effective teamwork. Carson, Tesluk, and Marrone (2007) suggested that collaborative leadership is enacted within two forms: focused and distributed. "Focused leadership occurs when leadership resides within a single individual, whereas distributed leadership occurs when two or more individuals share the roles, responsibilities, and functions of leadership" (Carson et al., 2007, p. 1218). Collaborative or shared leadership is usually supported through a formal organizational leader referred to by Pearce and Sims (2002) as the vertical leader. The collaborative team then interacts with the vertical leader to ensure the teamwork 'fits' within the overall organization. Orchard and Rykhoff (2015) proposed a complementary leadership framework that combines Pearce and Sims's concepts of vertical and shared leadership, which are integrated through a reciprocal building of relationships between the vertical leader's transformative, transactional, and empowering leadership (Pearce & Barkus, 2004), and the team members' shared leadership connected by shared relational coordination, as proposed by Gittell, Godfrey, and Thistlethwaite (2013). Both the vertical leader and the team in their shared leadership adopt the transformative leadership elements, advocated by Kouzes and Posner (2012), to (a) "model the way" (p. 16) or clarify each other's values and validate and connect actions to the team's shared values; (b) "inspire a shared vision" (p. 17) or help the team to see a desired future; (c) "enable others to act" (p. 21) or seek opportunities for both the manager and the team to innovate and take risks; (d) "challenge the process" (p. 19) or seek innovative ways to change, grow, and inspire; and (e) "encourage the heart" (p. 23) or recognize contributions of each other and the team together. When the shared leadership elements are operationalized in practice, there is a greater likelihood that the competency of collaborative or shared leadership will be demonstrated.

Samara reflected on how she was sharing in the leadership within the small team when she organized a meeting with their new patient Philip. She realized that she had taken control of the situation and seemed to be operating more in an independent than a shared approach. She also thought about how she had approached Philip and felt she needed to work on how to make her clients feel that they were the 'controllers' of their care. She wrote a note to herself that on Philip's next visit to their team she needed to have him determine more about what he really wanted to work on to help support his management of his diabetes. Samara also remembered that at one point in the team meeting with Philip that the dietitian disagreed with Samara's suggestion about how Philip needed to adjust his diet. She realized that she ignored this comment and really needed to be more open to learning how to work through such disagreements. Philomena really has much more knowledge about diet than she does, and Samara needs to let her know she values her input. Samara realized that Philip's treatment team needs to have a process to work through any disagreements.

Interprofessional Conflict Resolution

How people react to disagreements or conflict situations is dependent on their "relationship within the team (power dynamics); the situation the team is addressing; how other people in the team respond; and whether members are seeking to achieve their own personal or the team's goal" (Adler & Proctor, 2010, p. 347). Key interprofessional team working skill development should focus on each member's capacity to negotiate and work toward collaborative decision making. While conflicts are often perceived as 'troublesome' by other health providers, they are actually healthy and allow for a variety of perspectives to be shared, and, when handled well, can result in high quality comprehensive and collaborative patient care planning. The goal in interprofessional conflict resolution is finding a win-win solution to any team disagreement. Sexton (2014) conducted a survey of health educators and practitioners and found only 30% of the respondents ($n = 160$) reported having received any training in conflict resolution. Zweibel, Goldstein, Manwaring, and Marks (2008) reported on conflict resolution training provided to medical residents and academic health care faculty at two universities in Canada. The workshop was 2 days in length and focused on an integrated framework from scholars in the area. The framework is comprised of four components: (a) "identifying sources of conflict and conflict management roles" (Zweibel et al., 2008, p. 323); (b) "uncovering the needs and concerns, referred to as interests, that motivate the demands or positions taken by people in conflict" (p. 323); (c) "recognizing the impact of culture on how people define and handle conflict" (p. 323); and (d) applying communication skills" (p. 323). The framework is enacted through small group work, including role playing and facilitated discussions. In a post-workshop follow-up session authors reported "the pedagogical approach of using a conflict resolution framework as a guide for self-reflection, inquiry, preparation, and analysis worked well to prepare professionals for managing conflict in diverse workplace situations" (Zweibel et al., 2008, p. 345). However, this program was carried out with only one profession involved in the learning. Transferring this framework into a wider application has merit. However, the cost of releasing health providers for a full 2 days may not be always feasible. Another approach can be in guiding teams to use a process for resolution of their conflicts. A potential process, which has been used with positive evaluations in collaborative team-building 1-day workshops, is provided below:

- Create an openness to hear others views.
- Consider all views within your own perspective.
- Consider biases that might exist in your viewpoint.
- Consider justification for your biases and how you can come to terms with others views.
- Weight the alteration in your view, based on others views in the contest of the client's safety.
- Share your thinking with the other team members.
- Hear each other's viewpoints.
- Come to a shared agreement. (Orchard, 2014, pp. 48–49)

Samara remembered attending a student workshop on interprofessional conflict resolution and recalled that in any disagreement it is important to assume that different viewpoints from one's own always have some substantive value to the discussion. Therefore, by carefully listening to all the viewpoints expressed in the team and considering these against your own viewpoint provides a more robust perspective on how to address care that as an individual you may not have considered. Hence, using such a process is more likely to result in better care decisions than when health care practitioners make decisions by themselves.

CONCLUSION

In this chapter, the concept of competence and its associated competency and competencies have been explored within the context of interprofessional client-centered collaborative practice. Several approaches to how competence can be viewed were discussed, including skill based, life-skills based, behavior based, and finally an integrated approach.

Discussion of the application of capability frameworks was also addressed. Finally, the CIHC (2012) *Interprofessional Competency Framework* was discussed as a means to explore how collaboration as a process can be demonstrated. Throughout this chapter, a case study was used to illustrate how Samara, a young family practice resident, interacted with the elements to show how these apply to her practice within a primary care family practice unit.

REFERENCES

Adams, T. L., Orchard, C., Houghton, P., & Ogrin, R. (2014). The metamorphosis of a collaborative team: From creation to operation. *Journal of Interprofessional Care, 28,* 339–344. http://dx.doi.org/10.3109/ 13561820.2014.891571.

Adler, R. B., & Proctor, R. F., II. (2010). *Looking out looking in* (13th ed.). Boston, MA: Wadsworth Cengage Learning.

American Interprofessional Education Collaborative. (2011, May). *Core competencies for interprofessional collaborative practice.* Retrieved from http://www.aacn.nche.edu/ education-resources/ipecreport.pdf

Arford, P. H., & Zone-Smith, L. (2005). Organizational commitment to professional practice models. *Journal of Nursing Administration, 35,* 467–472. http://dx.doi.org/10.1097/ 00005110-200510000-00008.

Baker, G. R., Norton, P. G., Flintoft, V., Blais, R., Brown, A., Cox, J., ... Tamblyn, R. (2004). The Canadian adverse events study: The incidence of adverse events among hospital patients in Canada. *Canadian Medical Association Journal, 170,* 1678–1686. http://dx.doi.org/10.1503/ cmaj.1040498.

Canadian Interprofessional Health Collaborative. (2010, February). *A national interprofessional competency framework.* Retrieved from http://www.cihc.ca/files/ CIHC_IPCompetencies_Feb1210.pdf

Carson, J. B., Tesluk, P. E., & Marrone, J. A. (2007). Shared leadership in teams: An investigation of antecedent conditions and performance. *Academy of Management Journal, 50,* 1217–1234. http://dx.doi.org/10.2307/AMJ.2007.20159921.

Cheetham, G., & Chivers, G. (1996). Towards a holistic model of professional competence. *Journal of European Industrial Training, 20*(5), 20–30. http://dx.doi.org/ 10.1108/03090599610119692.

Conn, L. G., Lingard, L., Reeves, S., Miller, K. L., Russell, A., & Zwarenstein, M. (2009). Communication channels in general internal medicine: A description of baseline patterns for improved interprofessional collaboration. *Qualitative Health Research, 19,* 943–953. http://dx.doi.org/10.1177/1049732309338282.

Costa, A. C. (2003). Work team trust and effectiveness. *Personnel Review, 32,* 605–622. http://dx.doi.org/10.1108/00483480310488360.

Deneckere, S., Robyns, N., Vanhaecht, K., Euwema, M., Panella, M., Lodewijckx, C., ... Sermeus, W. (2011). Indicators for follow-up of multidisciplinary teamwork in care processes: Results of an international expert panel. *Evaluation & the Health Professions, 34,* 258–277. http://dx.doi.org/10.1177/0163278710393736.

Derouen, C., & Kleiner, B. H. (1994). New developments in employee training. *Work Study, 43*(2), 13–16. http://dx.doi.org/10.1108/ EUM0000000004315.

Epstein, R. M., & Hundert, E. M. (2002). Defining and assessing professional competence. *Journal of American Medical Association, 287*, 226–235. http://dx.doi.org/10.1001/jama.287.2.226.

Erdem, F., & Ozen, J. (2003). Cognitive and affective dimensions of trust in developing team performance. *Team Performance Management, 9*(5/6), 131–135. http://dx.doi.org/10.1108/13527590310493846.

Frank, J. R., Snell, L., & Sherbino, J. (Eds.). (2015, March). *The draft CanMEDS 2015: Physician competency framework*. Retrieved from http://www.royalcollege.ca/portal/page/portal/rc/common/documents/canmeds/framework/canmeds2015_framework_series _IV_e.pdf

Frank, J. R., Snell, L. S., Ten Cate, O., Holmboe, E. S., Carraccio, C., Swing, S. R., ... Harris, K. A. (2010). Competency-based medical education: Theory to practice. *Medical Teacher, 32*, 638–645. http://dx.doi.org/10.3109/0142159x.2010.501190.

Fraser, S. W., & Greenhalgh, T. (2001). Complexity science: Coping with complexity: Educating for capability. *British Medical Journal, 323*, 799–803. http://dx.doi.org/10.1136/bmj.323.7316.799.

Garavan, T. N., & McGuire, D. (2001). Competencies and workplace learning: Some reflections on the rhetoric and the reality. *Journal of Workplace Learning, 13*, 144–164. http://dx.doi.org/10.1108/13665620110391097.

Gittell, J. H., Godfrey, M., & Thistlethwaite, J. (2013). Interprofessional collaborative practice and relational coordination: Improving healthcare through relationships. *Journal of Interprofessional Care, 27*, 210–213. http://dx.doi.org/10.3109/13561820.2012.730564.

Greenhalgh, T., & Macfarlane, F. (1997). Towards a competency grid for evidence-based practice. *Journal of Evaluation in Clinical Practice, 3*, 161–165. http://dx.doi.org/10.1046/j.1365-2753.1997.00082.x.

Grzeda, M. M. (2005). In competence we trust? Addressing conceptual ambiguity. *Journal of Management Development, 24*, 530–545. http://dx.doi.org/10.1108/02621710510600982.

Hackett, S. (2001). Educating for competence and reflective practice: Fostering a conjoint approach in education and training. *Journal of Workplace Learning, 13*, 103–112. http://dx.doi.org/10.1108/ 13665620110388406.

Hibbard, J. H., Mahoney, E. R., Stock, R., & Tusler, M. (2007). Do increases in patient activation result in improved self-management behaviors? *Health Services Research, 42*, 1443–1463. http://dx.doi.org/10.1111/ j.1475-6773.2006.00669.x.

Howarth, M., Warner, H., & Haigh, C. (2012). "Let's stick together" – a grounded theory exploration of interprofessional working used to provide person centred chronic back pain services. *Journal of Interprofessional Care, 26*, 491–496. http://dx.doi.org/10.3109/ 13561820.2012.711385

Institute of Medicine. (2001, March). *Crossing the quality chasm: A new health system for the 21st century*. Retrieved from https://www.iom.edu/~/media/Files/Report%20Files/2001/Crossing-the-Quality-Chasm/Quality%20Chasm%202001%20%20report%20brief.pdf

Khomeiran, R. T., Yekta, Z. P., Kiger, A. M., & Ahmadi, F. (2006). Professional competence: Factors descried by nurses as influencing their development. *International Nursing Review, 53*, 66–72. http://dx.doi.org/10.1111/j.1466-7657.2006.00432.x.

Kouzes, J. M., & Posner, B. Z. (2012). The leadership challenge: How to make extraordinary things happen in organizations (5th Ed.). San Francisco, CA: Jossey-Bass.

Le Deist, F. D., & Winterton, J. (2005). What is competence? *Human Resource Development International, 8*(1), 27–46. http://dx.doi.org/ 10.1080/1367886042000338227.

Lee, H.-J. (2004). The role of competence-based trust and organizational identification in continuous improvement. *Journal of Management Psychology, 19,* 623–639. http://dx.doi.org/10.1108/02683940410551525.

Macdonald, M. B., Bally, J. M., Ferguson, L. M., Lee Murray, B., Fowler-Kerry, S. E., & Anonson, J. M. S. (2010). Knowledge of the professional role of others: A key interprofessional competency. *Nurse Education in Practice, 10,* 238–242. http://dx.doi.org/10.1016/j.nepr.2009.11.012.

Mansfield, R. (2004). Competence in transition. *Journal of European Industrial Training, 28,* 296–309. http://dx.doi.org/10.1108/ 030905904105276672.

McNair, R. P. (2005). The case for educating health care students in professionalism as the core content of interprofessional education. *Medical Education, 39,* 456–464. http://dx.doi.org/10.1111/j.1365-2929.2005.02116.x.

Moore, D. R., Cheng, M.-I., & Dainty, A. R. J. (2002). Competence, competency and competencies: Performance assessment in organisations. *Work Study, 51,* 314–319. http://dx.doi.org/10.1108/00438020210441876.

Orchard, C. A. (2009, July 30). Patient centred collaborative care [Video file]. Retrieved from https://www.youtube.com/watch?v=h7jHp5ooNec.

Orchard, C. A. (2014). TEAMc –Toolkit to enhance and assist maximizing team collaboration facilitator workbook. London, Ontario: Western University.

Orchard, C. A., Curran, V., & Kabene, S. (2005). Creating a culture for interdisciplinary collaborative practice. *Medical Education Online, 10*(11), 1–13. Retrieved from http://www.med-ed-online.net/index.php/ meo/article/viewFile/4387/4569.

Orchard, C. A., & Rykhoff, M. (2015). Collaborative leadership within interprofessional practice. In D. Forman, M. Jones, & J. Thistlethwaite (Eds.), *Leadership and collaboration: Further developments for interprofessional education, (pp. 71-94).* Basingstoke, United Kingdom: Palgrave MacMillan.

Pearce, C. L., & Barkus, B. (2004). The future of leadership: Combining vertical and shared leadership to transform knowledge work. *The Academy of Management Executive, 18*(1), 47–57.

Pearce, C. L., & Sims, H. P., Jr. (2002). Vertical versus shared leadership as predictors of the effectiveness of change management teams: An examination of aversive, directive, transactional, transformational, and empowering leader behaviors. *Group Dynamics: Theory, Research, & Practice, 6,* 172–197. http://dx.doi.org/10.1037//1089-2699.6.2.172.

Reeves, S., Fox, A., & Hodges, B. D. (2009). The competency movement in the health professions: Ensuring consistent standards or reproducing conventional domains of practice? *Advanced in Health Science Education, 14,* 451–453. http://dx.doi.org/10.1007/s10459-009-9166-2.

Robinson, F. P., Gorman, G., Slimmer, L. W., & Yudkowsky, R. (2010). Perceptions of effective and ineffective nurse–physician communication in hospitals. *Nursing Forum, 45,* 206–216. http://dx.doi.org/10.1111/j.1744-6198.2010.00182.x.

Roegiers, X. (2007). Curricular reforms guide schools: But, where to? *Prospects, 37,* 155–186. http://dx.doi.org/10.1007/s11125-007-9024-z.

Salas, E., DiazGranados, D., Weaver, S. J., & King, H. (2008). Does team training work?: Principles for health care. *Academic Emergency Medicine, 15*(11), 1002–1009. http://dx.doi.org/10.1111/j.1553-2712.2008.00254.x.

Sexton, M. E. (2014). *Determinants of healthcare professionals' self-efficacy to resolve conflicts that occur among interprofessional collaborative teams* (Doctoral dissertation). Retrieved from http://rave.ohiolink.edu/etdc/view?acc_num=toledo1396104234.

Stoof, A., Martens, R. L., van Merriënboer, J. J. G., & Bastiaens, T. J. (2002). The boundary approach of competence: A constructivist aid for understanding and using the concept of competence. *Human Resource Development Review, 1*, 345–365. http://dx.doi.org/10.1177/1534484302013005

Suter, E., Arndt, J., Arthur, N., Parboosingh, J., Taylor, E., & Deutschlander, S. (2009). Role understanding and effective communication as core competencies for collaborative practice. *Journal of Interprofessional Care, 23*, 41–51. http://dx.doi.org/10.1080/13561820802338579.

Tardif, J. (1999). *Le transfers des apprentissages* [Transfer of learning]. Montréal, Canada: Les Éditions Logiques.

ten Cate, O., & Scheele, F. (2007). Competency-based postgraduate training: Can we bridge the gap between theory and clinical practice? *Academic Medicine, 82*, 542–547. http://dx.doi.org/10.1097/ ACM.0b013e31805559c7

Travis, J. (2002). Cross-disciplinary competency standards for work-related assessments: Communicating the requirements for effective professional practice. *Work, 19*, 269–280.

University of Western Ontario, Office of the Interprofessional Health Education & Research. (2014). *Patient/client*. Retrieved from http://www.ipe.uwo.ca/Professionals/patient.html

Walsh, C. L., Gordon, M. F., Marshall, M., Wilson, F., & Hunt, T. (2005). Interprofessional capability: A developing framework for interprofessional education. *Nurse Education in Practice, 5*, 230–237. http://dx.doi.org/10.1016/j.nepr.2004.12.004.

West, M. A., & Field, R. (1995). Teamwork in primary health care. 1: Perspectives from organizational psychology. *Journal of Interprofessional Care, 9*, 117–122. http://dx.doi.org/10.3109/13561829509047845.

Zweibel, E. B., Goldstein, R., Manwaring, J. A., & Marks, M. B. (2008). What sticks: How medical residents and academic health care faculty transfer conflict resolution training from the workshop to the workplace. *Conflict Resolution Quarterly, 25*, 321–350. http://dx.doi.org/10.1002/crq.211.

In: Interprofessional Client-Centred Collaborative Practice
ISBN: 978-1-63483-754-5
Editor: Carole Orchard
© 2015 Nova Science Publishers, Inc.

Chapter 3

PERIOPERATIVE PRACTICE IN THE CONTEXT OF CLIENT-CENTERED CARE

Marion Jones[1], Isabel Jamieson[2] and Leigh Anderson[3]

[1]Auckland University of Technology, Auckland, New Zealand
[2]Christchurch Polytechnic Institute of Technology,
Christchurch, New Zealand
[3]Auckland District Health Board, Auckland, New Zealand

ABSTRACT

This chapter focuses on perioperative practice in the context of client-centered care presented as a case study set within the New Zealand Health Care System. It demonstrates how a perioperative team worked together to contribute to the best outcome for Mr. Stanley (pseudonym). Orchard, Curran, and Kabene's (2005) conceptual model for patient-centered care is used as a framework to interpret the case study. This model allows consideration of the decision-making processes within the organization to highlight the power imbalances between health professionals and the resultant behaviors exhibited. Examination of Mr. Stanley's case study provides the map for how interprofessional client-centered care should happen for a positive outcome for all team members.

INTRODUCTION

Collaborative practice requires not only the interprofessional team to work together but also requires a cultural change to move from uni-professionism to interprofessionalism. Given the importance of ensuring the best possible client outcomes and to enhance interprofessional practice, client-centered care and collaborative practice needs to occur in the perioperative context. Nursing, medical, and allied health teams must work alongside each other in order to safely and effectively deliver care. Davis (2009) cautions, "Modern surgery is so complex that it is beyond the ability of any profession, or professional group, to assure safety and quality in an absolute sense ... [therefore] we need higher levels of teamwork and communication" (p. 24).

INTERPROFESSIONAL COLLABORATIVE PRACTICE IN THE OPERATING THEATER

The World Health Organization (WHO) views "interprofessional collaboration in education and practice as an innovative strategy that will play an important role in mitigation in the global workforce crisis" (World Health Organization [WHO], 2010, p.7). WHO (2010) goes on to suggest that collaborative practice occurs when health care personnel from different disciplines work together to offer the best possible care to patients, their families, and communities. Given the WHO concerns regarding the importance of interprofessional practice and the increasing acuity of patients coupled with the more complex procedures, complex systems, and the highly technical nature of surgical work in the operating room, it is timely to make transparent the importance of interprofessional collaboration in the operating theater.

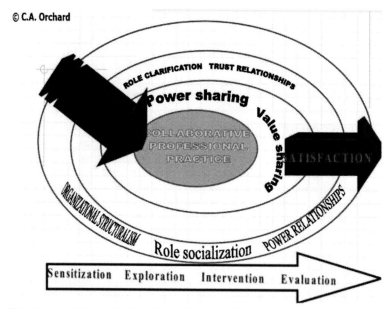

Note. From "Creating a Culture for Interdisciplinary Collaborative Professional Practice," by C. A. Orchard, V. Curran, & S. Kabene, 2005, *Medical Education Online, 10,* p. 2. Copyright 2005 by Orchard et al., Reprinted with permission.

Figure II. Creating a Culture for Interdisciplinary Collaborative Professional Practice.

Bleakley, Boyden, Hobbs, Walsh and Allard (2006) note that operating theater teams may exhibit multi-professional behavior, rather than interprofessional practice, whereas the context is ripe for interprofessional practice. Orchard et al., (2005) emphasize the importance of the processes teams go through to develop collaborative practice. The following case study, set in the New Zealand health care system, will demonstrate how a perioperative team worked together to contribute to the best outcome for this client. The case study will be interpreted in sections identifying the collaborative processes using Orchard et al.'s conceptual model for client-centered care (see Figure III).

The goal within this model is to recognize how important it is to consider not only the decision-making processes within the organization, but also to demonstrate the power imbalances between health professionals and the resultant behaviors exhibited. For the purpose of this chapter, the perioperative period starts at the time that a decision is made to perform surgery (pre-assessment admission to hospital) and finishes when the patient is discharged from the hospital and referred back to the care of the general practitioner (GP).

CASE STUDY

The aim of Orchard et al.'s (2005) model (see Figure II) is to transform any of the barriers of client-centered care into enablers so as to promote interprofessional team practice. This case outlines Mr. Stanley's journey through the perioperative experience process and the overall reflections on the client-centered care undertaken. In this chapter pseudonyms have been used to conceal all identities.

Pre-Operative Phase

Mr. Stanley is a 66-year-old retired forklift driver who has lived alone since his divorce 20 years ago. He has one adult daughter, Diana, who lives close by. However, he doesn't see her very often. His relationship with his family has never been an easy one due to his behavior while addicted to drugs and alcohol in his younger years. As a result, Mr. Stanley contracted Hepatitis C from sharing needles. Since this time he has overcome an addiction to drugs and alcohol and become sober.

Recently, at a routine health check with his GP, Mr. Stanley was diagnosed as having Hepatocellular Carcinoma. Mr. Stanley reached out to his daughter for support. They were both alarmed and anxious about the diagnosis and had many questions. Mr. Stanley was referred to the local public hospital's surgical team for surgery. Prior to surgery Diana took her father to the hospital to meet with the initial team that would be involved with his care. They were very surprised that instead of just meeting the surgeon there was a team of people who were there to discuss his care with him. At the meeting were the surgeon, anesthetist, nurse specialist, and a social worker. The surgeon proposed a plan of care, which was discussed and then Mr. Stanley was able to ask questions and talk about his concerns. He was happy to have the surgery but was scared about what would happen afterwards, as he lived alone and had nobody to help him. The social worker offered several solutions to assist, and they agreed that she would visit him at home in the next few days so that they could work through his specific issues. Once all concerns were discussed, the need for a written surgical consent was explained and then signed by both parties. Diana voiced her fear that she "didn't want the same thing to happen to her Dad that happened to her Great Uncle Tony when he had his operation." She explained that her grandfather always used to talk about how Tony went in to the operating room for a routine operation and died of an allergic reaction that made his temperature go very high. These comments triggered an alarm with the anesthetist who was considering the possibility of Mr. Stanley being at risk of Malignant Hyperthermia (MH). The decision was made to schedule him first on the list to minimize the exposure to MH trigger agents. The anesthetist also discussed pain relief options, explaining that he recommended an intrathecal morphine injection immediately pre-operatively for optimal pain relief. He also reassured them both that intravenous pain relief would be available at any time. Mr. Stanley was also given a copy of the Patient Code of Rights pamphlet (Auckland District Health Board, 2014).

Mr. Stanley and his daughter were involved in this pre-operative discussion as the interprofessional team worked together to plan for his forthcoming surgery and recovery. Clear communication, role clarification, and power sharing were evident, demonstrating that members of the interprofessional team were willing and able to include the client and his significant other in the planning stage of the client's care. This process also highlighted how a potential problem (MH) may not have been discovered prior to the surgery if the daughter had not been part of the team discussion and the team's openness to listen to her.

On the afternoon prior to surgery, there was a routine strategic team meeting in the theater suite to plan the surgical lists for the following day. The theater nurse manager, specialist anesthetist coordinator, and nursing coordinator discussed the client load for the following day. The theater nurse manager brought up that a key concern for Mr. Stanley was his potential risk for MH. It was confirmed that he was first on the list and the coordinators agreed to discuss this case further with both the nursing and anesthetic teams to ensure the correct procedures were followed and also that all safety equipment was on hand and checked ready to be used should this be required. They agreed how to best communicate this safety concern so that all team members were aware of the risk for Mr. Stanley.

This discussion demonstrates how *organizational structuralism* allowed decision-making practices to be proactive and interprofessional. The *organizational structuralism* included clear documentation; safety, including cultural safety and trust relationships developing, along with evidence demonstrating power sharing; and valuing of each other's expertise. This recognizes the importance of building trust relationships not only with the client but also between the health professionals working within the team, thereby recognizing the balance of power needed along with role socialization.

After this meeting, Mr. Stanley underwent further tests and assessment to ensure that he was ready and in optimal condition for surgery. He was scheduled for a Tuesday morning surgery, and the nurse told him he should be at the hospital at 0630 without having anything to eat or drink.

On the morning of surgery, staff were busy planning and preparing for the day ahead. The team from Mr. Stanley's theater had their morning briefing. The anesthetist explained to the team Mr. Stanley's potential risk for MH. The anesthetic technician ran through the preparation of equipment that had occurred. The nurses in the team confirmed that they had the necessary emergency equipment on hand, and placed the contact numbers of those who would assist, if required, written prominently on the whiteboard and as well as programed into the theater phones. The team agreed that they were prepared to deal with a MH emergency and would take every precaution to avoid an allergic reaction but were prepared to act should anything happen.

Exploration of Mr. Stanley's status to be in an optimal health condition for surgery was undertaken through the leadership of the surgeon and the health professional team present.

This included the clinical nurse specialist working with other key team members (i.e., the laboratory technician, radiographer, and social worker). Orchard et al., (2005) stress that collaboration is based on a relationship of interdependence built on respect, trust, and understanding of the unique and complementary perspectives of each profession (p. 5). When this is evident, resolution of the power imbalances result along with transparency of practice within the roles.

Meanwhile, Mr. Stanley and Diana arrived in the theater suite and were greeted by one of the nurses into the pre-operative department. Diana was told that she was welcome to stay with her father until he went into surgery. They both had last-minute questions answered by the pre-operative nurse. The importance of family and interprofessional leadership is critical when emphasizing client-centered care. Mr. Stanley's anesthetist and surgeon both came to see him to reassure him that all precautions had been taken to avoid any allergic reaction to the anesthetic agent. His pre-operative checklist was completed and paperwork finalized. When the time came for Mr. Stanley to go through to the theater (Operating Room) he said farewell to his daughter. The theater nurse checked his bracelet and confirmed all the details. On the way to theater she made reference to the Surgical Safety Checklist and that there would be one more check of his details before he was anesthetized. He expressed to the nurse that he was extremely nervous but confident in the team.

At this phase of the surgical journey Mr. Stanley meets more members of the interprofessional team and the handover process from the pre-operative nurse is critical to maintain continuity of care. The surgical safety check is formalized at this stage (WHO, 2008), with all the team members involved in the intra-operative phase being present, demonstrating working together in collaborative practice.

Clinicians engaging with and involving the client in planning his or her care can lead to improved health outcomes and a better use of health care services (Coulter & Ellins, 2006). In the operating theater this collaboration was evidenced by the use of the Surgical Safety Checklist (WHO, 2008). This tool is promoted by the WHO and has been adopted internationally and is shown to enhance interprofessional collaboration. This tool facilitates team conversations using a prescribed set of questions at key periods during the surgical procedure. These conversations prevent common errors from occurring that can lead to errors and a poor outcome for the client (WHO, 2008).

Intra-Operative Phase

As the theater doors opened the team focused on getting Mr. Stanley on to the theater bed and wrapped in a warmed blanket. He was welcomed by the anesthetist and the perioperative nurse. The anesthetist began the sign-in portion of the Surgical Safety Checklist (WHO, 2008) guided by the prompt card poster, and read aloud from the client identification bracelet for the team to hear and asked if it was correct. Mr. Stanley confirmed his name and also that he was there to have a liver resection. After this the team again had a brief discussion about the MH risk. This was to reassure Mr. Stanley that everyone knew about his potential risk. He appeared relaxed when he was anesthetized.

Prior to commencing surgery the nursing team members, anesthetist, surgeon, technician, and students present all completed the time-out phase of the WHO (2008) *Surgical Safety Checklist*. Once safely positioned, Mr. Stanley's 3-hour surgery proceeded as the team had planned. Mr. Stanley's vital signs were monitored constantly and showed no signs of MH at any stage.

The safety and monitoring required during this phase reinforces the need for interprofessional working to maintain an optimal health status for Mr. Stanley and demonstrates the critical importance of trusting relationships. Collaborative professional practice was led by the anesthetist and circulating nurse while keeping all other team members fully informed of the client's status along with important phases of the surgery itself.

Post-Operative Phase

Soon after Mr. Stanley arrived in the Post-Anesthetic Care Unit (PACU), Diana received a call that her father's surgery had been completed without complications. Monitoring of vital signs continued for 1.5 hours and his pain was managed. Before leaving PACU the pain team were called and they fine-tuned his pain relief as per the pre-operative discussions. A plan for ongoing pain management on the ward was agreed to, implemented, and documented. Mr. Stanley stayed in hospital for 6 days post-operatively; while on the ward, the wider team — physiotherapy and pharmacy — had input into his daily care.

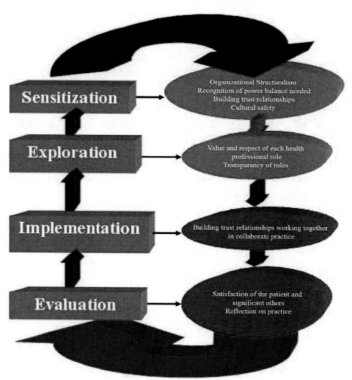

Note. Adapted from "Creating a Culture for Interdisciplinary Collaborative Professional Practice," by C. A. Orchard, V. Curran, & S. Kabene, 2005, *Medical Education Online, 10,* p. 3. Copyright 2005 by Orchard et al., Reprinted with permission.

Figure III. The process of the Interprofessional Team working with Mr. Stanley.

Mr. Stanley and his daughter were involved in developing his plan for discharge from hospital to ensure he was supported. This included scheduling visits from district nurses (home care nurses) to help with his dressing changes, assisted bathing, and arranging 'meals on wheels' to be delivered daily for the first 2 weeks. His care proceeded as per the plan, and Diana agreed to take him to his follow-up hospital appointments.

Mr. Stanley recovered well from his surgery and speaks highly of the team who took care of him and how he felted involved with his own care. He was also referred to the MH clinic for DNA testing and genetic counseling and was looking forward to finding out whether he actually is allergic to certain anesthetic agents.

The importance of the expansion of the interprofessional team at this phase is recognized as critical to meet the client needs and included a physiotherapist and pharmacist who conducted ongoing consultation and collaboration with Mr. Stanley and the family. With this extension of the interprofessional team, role clarification needed to be discussed to ensure each role is respected and valued in a client-centered care approach. This is moving the practice from the sensitization phase of the model to both the exploration and intervention stage (see Figure III). WHO (2010) emphasizes that to ensure future generations of health care providers collaborate effectively, we need to introduce opportunities for interprofessional learning and development that include learning "about, from and with each other" (p. 7).

DISCUSSION AND IMPLICATIONS

For effective interprofessional collaboration and the resultant changing context, the leadership needs to be safe, encouraging, and help each member of the team to succeed. Bass (1985) and Bass and Riggio (2006) emphasize the importance of transformational leadership in that members of the team need to be passionate and inspired along with feeling empowered through the leadership and team work that exists. Lamb and Clutton (2012) note that leadership for interprofessional teams is to drive improvement and patient safety, along with considering the stages of team development (Orchard et al., 2005; see Figure II).

Pre-Operative Phase of the Interprofessional Client-Centered Care Experience

In this case study, Mr. Stanley begins to experience interprofessional client-centered care at the pre-operative visit to the hospital when he was surprised that there were additional team members to the surgeon meeting with him. Initially, this was between the leader (the surgeon) and the followers (the nurse, anesthetist, social worker, the client, and his daughter). This provided the opportunity to not only set the scene for his surgical experience but also enabled the beginning of trust, safety, and communication relationships he needed, which inspires and empowers all the team members. This demonstrated the process of interprofessional collaboration , which reflected the trust and respect that comes through the sensitization phase of the client-centered care model (Orchard et al., 2005).

As noted by the Health Improvement and Innovation Resource Centre (2014), clear communication amongst the interprofessional team is of paramount importance, especially given that "research has shown that [poor] communication is a contributing factor to more than 60% of avoidable patient harm [occurrences]" (para. 4). It is vital that the interprofessional team set the scene of open communication early in the client encounter, as occurred in this instance, given that "tension spikes" (Lingard, Garwood, & Poenaru, 2004, p.692) may occur during the operative phase. According to Lingard et al., (2004), tension occurs in the perioperative setting when members of the interprofessional team have different views about the use of time, distribution, of resources and role clarification. As pressure increases to a point of a tension spike the outcome is that clear communication amongst the surgical team is hampered with potential for this to impact negatively on patient safety. In this case study, consideration was given to exploring each other's roles to give confidence to Mr. Stanley and show how each team member valued each other's contribution.

This experience continued into the immediate pre-operative period to follow the assumptions underpinning transformational leadership (Bass, 1985) in that the goals were focused on Mr. Stanley and the team and increasing their knowledge and awareness of the impending surgery. All team members were valued, thereby avoiding any threat that might occur across the professional boundaries.

Intra-Operative Phase of the Interprofessional Client-Centered Care Experience

Intra-operatively, the interprofessional team ensured Mr. Stanley was welcomed along with recognizing the importance of the WHO (2008) *Surgical Safety Checklist* being completed. Bass (1985) has used different components of transformational leadership, which include intellectual stimulation (the extent to which a leader will challenge assumptions); individualized consideration (the extent to which a leader addresses followers needs); and idealized influence (the charisma of a leader, which results in followers identifying with them). This clearly shows a new way to complete the checklist (intellectual stimulation) along with both providing support and encouragement (individualized consideration) and role modeling the process (idealized influence).

The role changes once Mr. Stanley is anesthetized, as the interprofessional team needs to act as an advocate and explore ways of working together to ensure the intra-operative phase is not elongated unnecessarily and communication channels are open and clear (providing examples of intellectual stimulation and individualized consideration). The role modeling of the leader is critical at this time, as the other members of the team need to trust, respect, and model the example set (providing an example of idealized influence). This also is the trusting relationship style needed in the implementation phase of Orchard et al.'s (2005) model.

Carney, West, Neily, Mills, and Bagian (2010) suggest that the different views expressed by profession groups about their perceptions of teamwork, especially the differences between perioperative nurses and surgeons, can hinder teamwork and emphasize the power imbalances. In this instance, it is clear that teamwork was enhanced. The ability to work together, as demonstrated in this case study, negates the view that "the surgical team does not always act as a cohesive team" (Rydenfält, Johansson, Larsson, Åkerman, & Odenrick, 2012, p. 792). Given that the key focus for the surgical team is client safety, it seems self-evident that an interprofessional approach to care delivery will be driven by the need to ensure the client's safety at all times (WHO, 2012). Furthermore, the collaboration of the interprofessional team is considered to be a vital contributing factor to the ongoing improvement of client outcomes (WHO, 2012).

Post-Operative Phase of the Interprofessional Client-Centered Care Experience

During the post-operative phase, Mr. Stanley assumes the role of a dependent person on the team while anesthetized and progressively moves to a person requiring assistance in the immediate and long-term recovery phase. As working together to focus on the interplay between pain management, wound care, and mobility assistance was required, the team needed to communicate clearly and share their observations and ensure his progress notes were available to all of the health professional team, providing an example of Bass's (1985) individualized motivation. Mr. Stanley's ongoing involvement in assessing his progress inspired Mr. Stanley to be motivated to achieve more each day, providing an example of Bass's (1985) inspirational motivation.

Questions asked of included how available were the relevant team members to him and his family, and did the communication demonstrate an effective interprofessional approach? He was involved in not only developing his discharge plan and follow-up hospital appointments but also felt involved with his own care, demonstrating client-centered and interprofessional working (see Figure IV– Implementation and Evaluation Phase).

Gilbert (2005) cautions that the lack of commitment from health professionals to deliver care using an interprofessional client-centered care approach may well result in situations in which "the patient/client [who] is compromised because of professional lack of understanding about the roles and responsibilities of fellow professionals" (p. 102).

Clinical and Administrative Responsibilities

The manager in each area is responsible for ensuring the pamphlets and posters outlining Code of Rights information are available for consumers and their families or whānau (a Māori term for extended family) and that local processes are in place for their distribution. Clinical teams are responsible to have in place clinical and administrative processes that support consumer rights, as outlined in the Code of Rights. Clinical staff are responsible for ensuring consumers are aware of the Code of Rights or similar codes in other countries and for providing the relevant written (pamphlets) and verbal information to consumers. Clinical documentation should include an appropriate application of these rights, for example providing written information given to consumers and families, use of interpreters, and involvement of support people. The Auckland District Health Board (2014), *Your Rights* pamphlet is based on the New Zealand Code of Health and Disability Services Consumers' Rights (1996) and also covers the Auckland District Health Board's complaints and privacy information. The pamphlet is also translated into a range of other languages (based on population information and interpreter usage) and includes the expectation, or responsibilities, Auckland District Health Board has of those receiving its services.

STRATEGIES TO ADDRESS CLIENT CASE ISSUES IN THE PERIOPERATIVE SETTING

The case study presented here is an actual account of a client's surgical experience explained against the backdrop of perioperative practice and the notion of interprofessional practice. While this case study highlights that interprofessional collaboration does occur throughout the client's journey, it is perhaps fair to say that this has occurred without any formal planning or organizational support. Furthermore, to our knowledge, no research has been undertaken in the New Zealand context to establish the efficacy of interprofessional collaboration with regard to better client outcomes. The following section offers some reflections and a range of strategies for consideration, which include interprofessional education, teamwork, and communication.

Establishing Continuing Interprofessional Education

Given the overwhelming evidence that the perioperative environment, especially the operating theater, is thwart with tension between interprofessionals (Coe & Gould, 2008; Lingard, Espin, et al., 2004; Lingard, Garwood, & Poenaru, 2004). It seems clear that formalized ongoing interprofessional education needs to occur so that health care teams can capitalize on promoting better client outcomes. Davis (2009) cautions, "Modern surgery is so complex that it is beyond the ability of any profession, or professional group, to assure safety and quality in an absolute sense... . [Therefore,] we need higher levels of teamwork and communication" (p. 24). Some time ago, Bleakley, Boyden, Hobbs, Walsh, and Allard (2006) noted that it was time to move from multi-professional behavior to interprofessional practice. In this case study, evaluation of client satisfaction was evident as Mr. Stanley planned with his daughter his ongoing care and follow-up hospital appointments.

Therefore, it is highly recommended that health care organizations incorporate the concept of ongoing interprofessional development into their strategic plans so that resources can be allocated to allow formal interprofessional education to be established. The underpinning concepts of interprofessional education — learning "about, from and with"— need to become 'business as usual' for all health care professionals (WHO, 2010, p.7). In their literature review of contemporary technical skills required for rapidly evolving surgical interventions, Healy, Undre, and Vincent (2006) note that interprofessional education has not been recognized as important. Hence opportunities to enhance effective teamwork have been compromised. However, emerging results from a pilot study in New Zealand involving 120 operating theater staff, known as Multidisciplinary Operating Room Simulation (MORSim) study, note that shorter hospital stays and reduced complication rates for clients may have been the outcome of this focused interprofessional education (Health Improvement and Innovation Resource Centre, 2014). This really emphasizes the need for a model of practice being used to provide the guide map for practice, and Orchard et al., (2005) provide that in their model (see Figure II).

To build on the success of such projects we suggest that educators from different disciplines form interprofessional education teams to develop and establish ongoing workplace interprofessional education programs and evaluation and auditing processes. We also recommend that the content of an interprofessional education program includes content about teamwork and communication.

Teamwork. A key concern reported in the literature involves the different views expressed by professional groups about their perceptions of teamwork, especially the differences between perioperative nurses and surgeons (Carney et al., 2010). Results from a survey undertaken with American perioperative nurses ($n = 378$) and surgeons ($n = 312$) using the Safety Attitudes Questionnaire (Sexton et al., 2006) noted that surgeons had a significantly more favorable perception than nurses regarding teamwork (Carney et al., 2010). Carney et al., speculate that this perceived difference can result in poor communication due to incorrect assumptions being made by both nurses and surgeons. Makary et al., (as cited in Carney et al., 2010) note, "Nurses are taught to communicate using the story of the patient, while physicians are trained to communicate using the headlines" (p. 726). Figure III identifies how a client-centered focus was undertaken for Mr. Stanley.

Other researchers such as Rydenfält et al., (2012) note that "the surgical team does not always act as a cohesive team" (p. 792). Their qualitative study of 15 Swedish health care professionals representing all members of the surgical team concluded that each subgroup of professionals (surgeons, anesthetists, anesthetic nurses, theater nurses, and assistant nurses) views the client differently. The result is that each subgroup works in parallel rather than as a cohesive team (Rydenfält et al., 2012). Rydenfält et al., theorized that this phenomena may go some way to explaining Lingard, Garwood, et al.'s (2004) findings of tension spikes and communication failures, whereas in this case study the team communication was demonstrated as part of the day-to-day practice.

Communication. Lingard, Garwood, et al., (2004) developed a research study with the aim of validating a theory of catalysts of tension in the operating theater. The inquiry consisted of a two-phased qualitative study conducted in Toronto, Canada, with a total of 43 operating theater personnel for Phase 1 involving focus groups and interviews (surgeons $n = 6$, nurses $n = 22$, anesthetists $n = 5$, trainees $n = 10$) and 45 for Phase 2 involving field observations (surgeons $n = 10$, nurses $n = 24$, anesthetists $n = 12$, trainees $n = 9$). A modified grounded theory approach was used to analyze data. Results noted that tension spikes due to communication issues were less evident in operating theater teams in smaller hospitals (Lingard, Garwood, et al., 2004). While teams in larger hospital settings (i.e., a large tertiary center) were likely to experience at least one high-tension event during all procedures, this was attributed to "the more intimate, family like atmosphere anecdotally ascribed to smaller institutions" (Lingard, Garwood, et al., 2004, p. 696).

Gardezi et al., (2009) note that nurses have often expressed that they feel inhibited in their abilities to communicate with doctors. Their study of communications between nurses and doctors, involving the observation of more than 700 surgical procedures over a 2-year period in three tertiary care hospitals in Toronto, Canada, revealed an unexpected finding — the phenomena of silence (Gardezi et al., 2009). Gardezi et al., rightly note that silence is an important factor in the operating theater setting. It contributes to safe practice and performance and may be indicative of an experienced theater team. However, in their study, while they recorded several instances of appropriate silences, they also noted instances of constrained silence whereby members of the theater team "remain silent when something of concern takes place" (Gardezi et al., 2009, p. 1393). Although these observed silences did not equate to client safety issues, Gardezi et al., argue that although such silences may be defensive or strategic, they are probably indicators of hidden factors. These factors maybe as far ranging from fear of revealing one's lack of knowledge to exposing the lack of skills of others. Regardless of the cause, Gardezi et al., rightly suggest that operating theater personnel need to be cognizant of the power of silences so that they better understand the complexities of interprofessional communications to promote a more harmonious working environment between the different professional groups. Gardezi et al., allude to the notion that a more harmonious working environment should enhance and encourage interprofessional collaboration, which in turn should contribute to the best outcomes for clients. Gillespie and Hamlin's (2009) literature synthesis of 21 research papers about the competence of perioperative nurses highlighted that, in order to be competent, these nurses need to be able to "adeptly manage myriad personalities and interpret verbal and nonverbal nuances" (p. 255). Based on the research studies they reviewed, Gillespie and Hamlin present a strong argument that a key role for perioperative nurses is to contribute to effective communication to mitigate adverse risk, with the ultimate aim of increasing client safety.

Another aspect of communications in the operating theater is the hesitance of health care personnel to challenge others who are seen as higher in the hierarchy. This reluctance to speak up may detract from creating a safe client environment, which arguably should be of paramount importance to all theater staff (Johnson & Kimsey, 2012).

Johnson and Kimsey (2012) demonstrated that interprofessional education sessions attended by theater personnel (n = 800+) from the Leigh Valley Health Network in Pennsylvania, USA, to promote a culture of safety can successfully change attitudes, increase one's understanding of others' roles, and highlight the need to challenge those in authority, especially when client safety is at risk. Interprofessional team debriefing sessions are recommended along with professional development workshops for all the team members, with emphasis on the stages of Orchard et al.'s (2005) model and the interprofessional client-centered practice employed with Mr. Stanley.

CONCLUSION

To consciously change practice, as outlined by Orchard et al.'s (2005) client-centered care model, health care professionals must create the need for change as well as challenge the assumptions of the role of key players — the health professionals, the client, and the client's family. In so doing, health professionals will be truly able to learn "about, from and with" (WHO, 2010, p. 7) each other and their clients.

This then empowers all team members to work with each other with the client as a focus. As Jones (2000) emphasizes, to shape interprofessional practice of the future, disciplines can no longer work alone and remain effective within the health care system. Jones goes on to say that the capabilities for team development and interprofessional practice include effective communication, adaptation to change, team development, and valuing difference, which concurs with the strategies recommended above. Mr. Stanley's case study provides the map for how interprofessional client-centered care should happen for a positive outcome for all team members.

REFERENCES

Auckland District Health Board. (2014). *"Your Rights" pamphlet CC1040 (and translations)*. Auckland, New Zealand: Author.

Bass, B. M. (1985). *Leadership and performance*. New York, NY: Free Press.

Bass, B. M., & Riggio, R. E. (2006). *Transformational leadership* (2nd ed.). New York, NY: Routledge.

Bleakley, A., Boyden, J., Hobbs, A., Walsh, L., & Allard, J. (2006). Improving teamwork climate in operating theatres: The shift from multiprofessionalism to interprofessionalism. *Journal of Interprofessional Care, 20*, 461–470. http://dx.doi.org/10.1080/13561820600921915.

Carney, B. T., West, P., Neily, J., Mills, P. D., & Bagian, J. P. (2010). Differences in nurse and surgeon perceptions of teamwork: Implications for use of a briefing checklist in the OR. *AORN Journal, 91*, 722–729. http://dx.doi.org/10.1016/j.aorn.2009.11.066.

Coe, R., & Gould, D. (2008). Disagreement and aggression in the operating theatre. *Journal of Advanced Nursing, 61*, 609–618. http://dx.doi.org/10.1111/j.1365-2648.2007.04544.x.

Coulter & Ellins (2006). *The Quality enhancing interventions project: Patient-focused interventions*. The Health Foundation. London.

Davis, C. (2009). Team health and safety. *Nursing Standard, 24*(2), 24–25.

Gardezi, F., Lingard, L., Espin, S., Whyte, S., Orser, B., & Baker, G. R. (2009). Silence, power and communication in the operating room. *Journal of Advanced Nursing, 65*, 1390–1399. http://dx.doi.org/10.1111/j.1365-2648.2009.04994.x.

Gilbert, J. H. (2005). Interprofessional learning and higher education structural barriers. *Journal of Interprofessional Care, 19*(Suppl. 1), 87–106. http://dx.doi.org/10.1080/13561820500067132.

Gillespie, B. M., & Hamlin, L. (2009). A synthesis of the literature on "competence" as it applies to perioperative nursing. *AORN Journal, 90*, 245–252. http://dx.doi.org/10.1016/j.aorn.2009.07.011.

Healey, A. N., Undre, S., & Vincent, C. A. (2006). Defining the technical skills of teamwork in surgery. *Quality and Safety in Health Care, 15*, 231–234. http://dx.doi.org/10.1136/qshc.2005.017517.

Health Improvement and Innovation Resource Centre. (2014). *Patients may benefit from operating room team simulations*. Retrieved from http://www.hiirc.org.nz/page/50415/patients-may-benefit-from-operating-room/;jsessionid=A8221A35592C98810CE537957E428E50?contentType=27&section=13416.

Johnson, H. L., & Kimsey, D. (2012). Patient safety: Break the silence. *AORN Journal, 95*, 591–601. http://dx.doi.org/10.1016/j.aorn.2012.03.002.

Jones (2000). *Shaping Team Practice in the context of health reform: Challenges, Tensions and Benefits. Unpublished* PhD Thesis, Flinders University South Australia.

Lamb, B., and Clutton, N. (2012). Leadership Development for IP Teams to drive improvement and patient safety. In Leadership Development for Interprofessional Education and Collaborative Practice (Eds. by Forman, D., Jones, M. & Thistlethwaite, J. Palgrave UK.

Lingard, L., Espin, S., Whyte, S., Regehr, G., Baker, G. R., Reznick, R., ... Grober, E. (2004). Communication failures in the operating room: An observational classification of recurrent types and effects. *Quality & Safety in Health Care, 13,* 330–334. http://dx.doi.org/10.1136/ qshc.2003.008425.

Lingard, L., Garwood, S., & Poenaru, D. (2004). Tensions influencing operating room team function: Does institutional context make a difference? *Medical Education, 38,* 691–699. http://dx.doi.org/10.1111/ j.1365-2929.2004.01844.x.

New Zealand Code of Health and Disability Services Consumers' Rights. (1996). Retrieved from http://www.legislation.govt.nz/regulation/public/ 1996/0078/latest/DLM209085 .html

Orchard, C. A., Curran, V., & Kabene, S. (2005). Creating a culture for interdisciplinary collaborative professional practice. *Medical Education Online, 10,* 11. http://dx.doi.org/10.3402/meo.v10i.4387.

Rydenfält, C., Johansson, G., Larsson, P. A., Åkerman, K., & Odenrick, P. (2012). Social structures in the operating theatre: How contradicting rationalities and trust affect work. *Journal of Advanced Nursing, 68,* 783–795. http://dx.doi.org/10.1111/j.1365-2648.2011.05779.x.

World Health Organization. (2008, June). *Surgical safety checklist.* Retrieved from http://www.who.int/patientsafety/safesurgery/tools_resources/SSSL_ Checklist_finalJun08.pdf

World Health Organization. (2010). *Framework for action on interprofessional education and collaborative practice.* Retrieved from http://whqlibdoc.who.int/hq/2010/ WHO_HRH_HPN_10.3_eng.pdf?ua=1

In: Interprofessional Client-Centred Collaborative Practice   ISBN: 978-1-63483-754-5
Editor: Carole Orchard   © 2015 Nova Science Publishers, Inc.

Chapter 4

SHOULD THERE BE AN *"I"* IN TEAM?
A NEW PERSPECTIVE ON DEVELOPING
AND MAINTAINING COLLABORATIVE NETWORKS
IN HEALTH PROFESSIONAL CARE

Lesley Bainbridge and Glenn Regehr
University of British Columbia, Vancouver, BC, Canada

ABSTRACT

In this chapter the authors challenge the reader to re-think the predominant rhetoric about interprofessional collaboration. They argue that health professional education still tends to prepare practitioners to demonstrate profession-specific knowledge and skills. To change the collaborative practices of students requires changes within the workplace; as such, teaching health care providers to collaborate more effectively is necessary. The authors suggest the concept of collaborative networks among health professionals to deliver care and argue that individual skills in four areas are necessary: building social capital, perspective taking, negotiating priorities, and conflict management. They conclude by encouraging teaching of practitioners to acknowledge their individual roles as part of collaborative networks of health professionals for improved care delivery to clients and for effective role modeling for students learning about collaborative practice.

INTRODUCTION

Interprofessional collaboration has been defined as "a process of communication and decision making that enables the separate and shared knowledge and skills of health care providers to synergistically influence the patient care provided" (Way, Jones, & Busing, 2000, p. 3). For some time now, effective interprofessional collaboration (IPC) has been recognized by educators, policy makers, and practitioners as vital for a successful health care system. Patient safety research has demonstrated that the highest percentage of adverse events is caused by lack of communication and collaboration both within and across professions

(Baker et al., 2004). From the health human services literature, staff satisfaction, which translates into recruitment and retention, is closely linked to feeling valued as part of an effective team (Suter & Deutschlander, 2010). Given the predicted shortages of health professionals over the next few years (World Health Organization [WHO], 2010), recruitment and retention are important issues that may be addressed, at least in part, through improved collaboration. In addition, the cost of health care is rising in many countries to an unprecedented level (WHO, 2010) and effective collaboration is seen as a mechanism for increasing efficiencies in the system (Frenk et al., 2010). Moreover, reliance on a single provider as gatekeeper will not improve access to appropriate health care for clients (Frenk et al., 2010), leading to the emergence of constructs such as Family Health Teams and Community Health Centers that, in theory, rely on an interprofessional approach to care (Goldman, Meuser, Rogers, Lawrie, & Reeves, 2010).

Despite this, IPC is not a tradition for many disciplines and organizations in the health care system. Although for some it appears to be an intuitive skill, for many collaboration must be taught and rehearsed. In recognition of this need, interprofessional education (IPE) has become a major focus of attention in health care at both education and practice levels. IPE has been defined as "occasions when two or more professions learn with, from and about each other for the purpose of improving collaboration and quality of care" (Centre for the Advancement of Interprofessional Education, 2002, para. 3). For both students and practitioners alike, IPE is seen as the process by which we can train collaboration, and it is not a new concept. As far back as the 1960s, proponents of team-based care believed that students and practitioners must learn together if they are to work together (Szaz, 1968). However, it is only in the past decade that focused attention, including the provision of targeted resources, has been placed on IPE in pre- and post-licensure contexts.

Today, it is largely taken for granted that IPE is the solution to the problem of suboptimal IPC in health care and is becoming an explicit component of educational programs and continuing professional development around the world (Frenk et al., 2010). Yet, in its ongoing adoption and evolution, IPE is demonstrating itself to be a problem of its own.

From an outcomes perspective, IPE suffers from the same problem of role modeling and hidden curriculum issues that plague many efforts at addressing cultural change in health care (Gofton & Regehr, 2006; Hafferty, 1998). That is, we attempt to teach the value and skills of IPC, but we are aware that in practice there are many environments in which collaborative practice does not appear to be valued, much less enacted, and adoption of the suboptimal practices of the environment become the norm. All these problems emerge from the apparent conundrum that to change culture we must focus on teaching enactment of the new cultural norm, but in order to teach this norm we must first change the current culture to support our efforts and our messages (Holmes, Harris, Schwartz, & Regehr, 2014).

It is the very nature of a conundrum that it cannot be solved using the same logic and assumptions that generated it in the first place. It is our goal in this chapter, therefore, to re-examine some of the logic and assumptions that are built into our current constructions of IPE for students and practitioners as the solution to IPC. Bolden and Gosling (2006) suggested,

Like a musical refrain, competencies offer a repetitive "hook" that offers a sense of structure and consistency but also acts as an injunction that obliges us to refrain from further thematic development. Thus, the refrain encourages us to return to the same familiar melody rather than pursuing other avenues of thought and expression that might, from the point of melodic coherence, be considered a distraction. (p. 148)

In the context of IPE and associated competencies for IPC, the 'repeated refrain' reinforces a focus on group behaviors and may divert our attention from another lens for IPC that drills down into more subtle *individual* ways of thinking and being. That is, we focus our attention on collaboration as a collective process, typically identifiable as team-based care. As a result, our IPE efforts tend to focus on teaching students and practitioners to be effective members of collaborative teams. Consistent with models of IPC, there is an emphasis (albeit not exclusive focus) on skills of team function, collaborative leadership, and shared decision making, as well as concepts of patient-centered care and values-based practice (Canadian Interprofessional Health Collaborative, 2010).

Of course these skills and values are important, but as they are conceptualized in IPC models and taught in IPE curricula, they may be setting our students and practitioners up for failure. Taking such an approach may be preparing practitioners to be effectively collaborative participants in effectively collaborative teams, when we know that these teams do not consistently exhibit optimal levels of collaboration. Moreover, it may be idealizing how teams function, ignoring the competing demands on practitioners that will sometimes position other priorities as more important than collaboration in a given moment. As well, it may be over-representing the stability of the teams in which many health care providers function on a day-to-day basis, and perhaps emphasizes too strongly collaboration that occurs in co-located team-based care. We believe that this discrepancy between the ideal and simplified model of collaboration that is taught in the IPE context, and the reality that new health care providers face when entering the clinical domain may produce a sense of cynicism and futility that rapidly leads to a reproduction of the problem in these fresh graduates.

Our approach for the remainder of this chapter, therefore, is to shift the question of how to create effective collaborators away from the focus of how we can best teach our health care practitioners to join effectively collaborative health care teams in which all members hold the same IPC values and are motivated to collaborate. Instead, we explore the question of how we can prepare our practitioners to develop, nurture, and maintain effective collaborative networks in contexts that do not always promote or enable stable and effectively collaborative teams. We suspect that such skills might also apply to participation in highly collaborative teams; however, critically, we will not conceptualize these skills in a way that requires such teams to exist.

METHODS

The concepts that are explored in this chapter emerged from a series of conversations between the authors, and with others, about the current state of IPE and its apparently limited success. These conversations raised more questions than answers about how we teach, practice, and conceptualize collaboration in the health care environment. What emerged from these conversations, in addition to the constructions articulated in the introduction, was a set of domains (both concepts and skills) that seemed important for the process of building collaborative networks. It is not our contention that this list is comprehensive, but rather that it represents a set of examples that can form the core of a new approach to training for IPC. In particular, four domains emerged as a starting point for such an approach: building social capital, perspective taking, negotiating priorities, and conflict management. Other concepts that were explored but are not represented in this chapter included relationship building and rhetoric.

The University of British Columbia health and social sciences databases were searched for papers that linked to each domain. The search focused on papers and documents from 1990 onwards, unless they seemed seminal and long lasting. Abstracts were reviewed and filtered through the lens of (a) links to collaboration and the skills necessary to collaborate well and (b) links to possible education information for teaching collaboration. Keywords used in the search included collaboration; collaboration in health; perceptions and perspective taking; conflict resolution; negotiation, negotiating, and negotiating in health; as well as social capital.

Once the domains began to take shape, conversations with a wider audience began, and as people provided perspectives and asked questions, it became clear that this area of study resonated for people, reinforcing the need to pursue this alternative model of collaboration in health care. These additional conversations also allowed us to shape our own understandings of how these concepts related specifically to the health care context and how each added to the current understanding of collaboration as we were developing it.

RESULTS

Through reflection on many conversations and responses from conference participants, each domain has been refined. The following sections offer a summary of our explorations in each domain and include a brief description of how they might be relevant to health care collaboration.

Building Social Capital

A key concept in any social interaction is developing an understanding of social capital. In a highly simplified form, social capital might function similarly to the straight exchange found in other forms of capital: "I'll do this for you now, in the expectation that down the road you will return the favor." However, the notion of social capital is likely more valuable as a concept when it is understood in its more complex social construction. Social capital has been defined in many ways, but for the purposes of this chapter we will borrow the definition offered by Adler and Kwon (2002): "Social capital is the goodwill available to individuals or groups. Its source lies in the structure and content of the actors' social relations. Its effects flow from the information, influence, and solidarity it makes available to the actor" (p. 23).

By "goodwill," Adler and Kwon (2002) were referring to notions of trust, sympathy, and forgiveness. Such goodwill between people not only enables individuals to draw on the resources of others in order to accomplish goals, but also provides a social buffer that offers individuals the benefit of the doubt. Having this sort of trust in a relationship, for example, may mean that one need not provide a full explanation of one's motives for a request or a full justification of the claim of urgency for a given request; in this sense, a trust-based engagement is more efficient than forms of engagement that do not have such trust. In addition, however, this form of social capital can smooth out potentially awkward exchanges:

an encounter in which one might be unreflectively abrupt does not necessarily lead to the conclusion that one is rude or unfriendly, but rather might be interpreted as "having a bad day." Further, in such an exchange, the presence of social capital might allow the other individual to feel safe enough to check in about the exchange, thereby providing the opportunity to clarify the context of the abruptness and even apologize in the moment, in turn avoiding potential rifts in the professional relationship and perhaps even building further social capital.

This last example raises a key feature of social capital. It is not merely earned and spent by an individual, but is built in a relationship. As Coleman (1998) suggested, it is located not in the actors themselves, but in their relations with other actors. Thus, social capital is not a zero-sum game in which, in any given exchange, one person spends and the other earns. Rather, effective exchanges between individuals or members of a group often create social capital for all in the exchange, building collective goodwill. Social capital also requires maintenance — it grows with appropriate use. However, if neglected, the relationships cease to have meaning and lose their efficacy (Putnam, 1993, 1995). Social capital can depreciate through non-use or abuse. It takes mutual commitment and cooperation from both or all parties and can be seriously damaged by one defection — the relationship then dissolves, along with whatever social capital is contained. In today's vulnerable health care systems, the collective spirit of a team may also be destroyed through organizational realignment or other external operational decisions (Putnam, 1993, 1995). Thus, social capital is not something that should be taken for granted or assumed, but must be constantly nurtured and gauged.

It is also worth noting that while the concept of social capital can be described as a positive construct that informs the capacity of individuals to develop effective relationships, it is not without risks. Strong team relationships that develop over time may over embed an individual in the relationship, thus reducing the flow of new ideas as well as introducing parochialism and inertia (Putnam, 1993, 1995). Rivalry may also be an unintended consequence of developing social capital within teams, and the quid pro quo can become a burden of obligation or a competition for the most social capital with a concomitant risk of a sense of personal failure (Putnam, 1993, 1995). Moreover, Bordieu (1986) asserted that social capital is not merely contained to the capital built within a relationship; it can also be imbued though social structures in the form of institutionally derived power. Such externally imposed forms of social capital might be particularly prone to be used coercively to override others and to enforce social hierarchies.

Notwithstanding these cautions, the concept of social capital is one that lends itself well to the ability of individuals to create collaborative relationships and for generalized collectivity to "mak[e] possible the achievement of certain ends that in its absence would not be attainable" (Coleman, 1998, p. S98). Thus, teaching this concept to our students could offer them a vital tool for developing IPCs. If we can describe how the building of social capital is necessary as a primary skill for those who perform well in collaborative care contexts, we can teach students and practitioners to understand what they are actually doing when they engage in forms of social or professional exchange: they are not merely bartering for favors, but building goodwill within relationships and groups in order to contribute to the collective responsibility for effective collaborative patient-centered care.

Perspective Taking

Humans are natural inference makers. We are constantly developing stories and causal explanations to understand our world and the experiences we have in it. This extends to our interactions with others, in which we constantly attribute motivations to others' choices and actions (Boland & Tenkasi, 1995). Unfortunately, we usually do this based on our own perspective, with its limited representation of the world. As Schulz (2010) suggested, we are strongly motivated to see ourselves as "right," and as a consequence we tend to assume that our beliefs perfectly reflect reality. Thus, when others act in ways that are incompatible with our own sense of how that individual ought to act, we have a problem to solve: we must explain why they might have behaved differently than they "should" from our perspective. As Schulz (2010) argued, we tend to assume one of three things: that people are ignorant (they simply don't know the facts), they are idiots (they are too stupid to understand the situation), and they are evil (they are acting for their own malevolent purposes). Seldom, unfortunately, do we assume that others may have facts we do not or that they may have other equally valid goals for this situation that are not perfectly compatible with our own.

Thus, another vital concept that we must teach and reinforce is the skill of perspective taking — not just the *ability* to use it, but the *propensity* to use it. There are a number of documented positive consequences to the practice of perspective taking. According to several authors, actively instructing people to engage in perspective taking is associated with a variety of desirable effects, from inducing more favorable judgments of others (Epley, Keysar, Van Boven, & Gilovich, 2004), to increasing altruism and helping (Batson et al., 1991), to reducing stereotyping and prejudice (Galinsky & Moskowitz, 2000, 2001). In their article on perspective taking, Davis, Conklin, Smith, and Luce (1996) stated,

Both Mead (1934) and Piaget (1932) argued that possessing and using an ability to take another's perspective is responsible for much of human social capacity. According to this view, well-developed perspective-taking abilities allow us to overcome our usual egocentrism, tailor our behaviors to others' expectations, and thus make satisfying interpersonal relations possible. (p. 713)

According to Cialdini, Brown, Lewis, Luce, and Neuberg (1997), there are differences between imagining how another person feels and imagining how you would feel if you were in their position. Engaging in this process is a step in the development of empathy.

As with all humans, health care providers make assumptions about the knowledge, beliefs, and motives of others (Boland & Tenkasi, 1995). We tend not to check out those assumptions before making judgments and acting upon them. Checking out what others know or perceive is a key component of perspective taking (Bakhtin, 1981; Krauss & Fussell, 1991). In addition, part of the perspective-taking process requires imagining what the point of view of the other person or people may be (Brown, 1981). Valuing diversity of knowledge by enabling each type of expertise to make unique representations of their understandings and assisting people with different expertise to better recognize and accept the different ways of knowing of others are the foundation for perspective taking. It opens up opportunities for learning more about the other perspectives that are possible in the situation, which in turn affords better negotiation and problem solving. However, it also reduces the tendency to stereotype, thereby offering more opportunity for creating strong and meaningful relationships with other people. (It is important to note that the effort to reduce stereotyping may be at odds with some of the current practices in IPE such as role clarification, which might rapidly devolve to an assumption that one knows what others are supposed to do in highly stereotyped ways.)

Perspective taking, we believe, is a learnable skill; however, again, it is not just a matter of teaching the ability to use it, but also the propensity to use it. Providing learners with the opportunity to observe interactions that involve different perspectives may be one way of enabling practitioners to recognize that it is 'not all about them' and that people who are acting differently from their expectations may not be ignorant, stupid, or evil. Thus, coming to recognize and value when differing perspectives are arising should be an explicit learning objective and focus of teaching in any IPC training.

Negotiating Priorities and Resources

Our model of ideal health care teams often seems to start with the premise that we all have (or should have) the same goal — the best care for the patient. However, this is almost certainly a naïve construction of typical health care team interactions (Lingard, Espin, Evans, & Hawryluck, 2004). Even from an individual provider's perspective, there are multiple considerations that go into decisions regarding best care. Recognizing and resolving, or at least balancing, such considerations in a flexible way is a critical component of clinical reasoning. Therefore, it should not be surprising that for any given patient, there are likely different versions of 'best care,' depending on each provider's perspective. Moreover, the care of any given patient is embedded in the context of a larger health system that might introduce larger considerations and goals into each provider's construction of what is best in a given situation (Leung et al., 2012). As a result, effective negotiation regarding these various priorities and goals is yet another vital skill for effective collaborative care. The question remains, in collaborative practice models, just what do we mean by negotiation and what is involved?

In some contexts, negotiation is constructed as 'getting what you want' or 'getting the most you can' (such as negotiating one's salary). This version of negotiation might be considered a process of persuasion or influence. Manning and Robertson (2003a, 2003b) drew a distinction between influencing and negotiating and found that in the context of the workplace people use various combinations of six influencing strategies: reason, assertion, exchange, courting favor, coercion, and partnership. While Manning and Robertson suggested that in certain circumstances influencing may be more appropriate than negotiating, in the context of health care, treating negotiation primarily as influencing may well be suboptimal. If the influencer is always persuading to their perspective or opinion, the opportunity for negotiating and co-creating options is lost. In addition, the influencer becomes the 'winner' each time, losing the concept of reaching a mutually agreed-upon solution or decision. Perhaps a more desirable model of negotiation is the notion of consensus building — one in which the intent is to accommodate and manage differing interests, goals, and priorities effectively. With this approach the outcome of the negotiation is not the agreement of goals, but a plan that dynamically accommodates various priorities and perspectives.

There are many models of effective negotiation, but most appear to assume that negotiation is enacted as a formal process that will occur at a planned moment. Thus, these models include strategies such as preparing in advance, planning one's timing and location (which may be its own negotiation), 'opening strategies,' and similar notions. By contrast much of the negotiation in the health care context is likely to be more spontaneous and opportunistic. Such negotiations, often about moment-by-moment use of resources and commitment of energies, are much less idealistic than the theories would suggest. For example, Lingard, Espin, et al. (2004) described the "forces of ownership and trade [that] have a central role in the daily negotiations that constitute teamwork in the ICU setting" (p. R407). These authors went on to state,

When these forces are ignored – that is, perceived ownership is not attended to, or one commodity is not offered in trade for another – tensions accumulate and collaboration becomes sluggish. When these forces are accommodated – for example, competition for ownership of resources is anticipated, or requests are accompanied by offers of trade – the team members navigate their competing interests more smoothly to act effectively together. (Lingard, Espin, et al., 2004, p. R407)

Lingard, Espin, et al. (2004) additionally pointed out that the goals in the negotiation regarding a particular patient are not always exclusively about that patient. Rather, larger systemic issues are often at play (e.g., discharging one patient creates space for another). Failing to understand the potential for other (often legitimate) goals and considerations that might be at play in a negotiation will almost certainly lead to frustration and suboptimal resolution. Bringing these processes to the attention of our students and practitioners, helping them understand what is happening, and teaching them to participate in a manner that is functional within the system but that can move the system toward more collaborative processes seems more sensible than teaching them about idealized conditions that likely will not be relevant to their daily practices.

Managing Conflict

Conflict has been defined as "a process of social interaction involving a struggle over claims to resources, power and status, beliefs, and other preferences and desires (Appelbaum, Abdallah, & Shapiro, 1999, p. 63). In the context of collaborative practice, it seems inevitable that active conflict will lead to breakdown in communication and, therefore, to gaps in seamless patient care with adverse effects for the patient but also for the health care providers (Rogers & Lingard, 2006). Thus, much of the effort toward improving collaborative practice seems to be aimed at avoiding situations of conflict. Yet conflict is inevitable. Disagreements about medical care (Studdert, Burns, et al., 2003), management plans that deviate from approved hospital policy or procedures (Lingard, Garwood, & Poenaru, 2004; Prescott & Bown, 1985; Studdert, Mello, et al., 2003), interpersonal issues among members of the health care team (Rogers & Lingard, 2006, p. 569) and differing values held by different professional groups that constitute the team (Deutsch, 1994), have all been identified as sources of interprofessional conflict. In addition to efforts to create conditions that minimize the likelihood of conflict, therefore, it seems important to also train health care providers to manage conflict when it (inevitably) does arise.

Acknowledging this, some IPE courses include the skills of conflict resolution. However, the term 'conflict resolution' is one that implies the conflict involves a negative encounter rather than an opportunity for dialogue and conversation. Manning and Robertson (2004) have suggested the term 'conflict-handling' as a way to offer alternative interpretations of the concept. However, within this chapter, consistent with Thomas (1992), we use the term conflict management as a way of capturing this more constructive way of addressing conflict.

A first step in effective conflict management might be to acknowledge that there are different types of conflict. Several authors, for example, have distinguished between *task* conflict and *relationship* conflict (DeDreu & Weingart, 2003; Simons & Peterson, 2000). Task conflict is characterized by disagreement regarding different ideas about a task and how it might be completed, whereas relationship conflict is characterized by friction, frustration, and personality clashes within the group (Jehn, 1994). These types of conflict are likely addressed in different ways, with task conflict likely being resolved with negotiation, but relational conflict requiring more interpersonal models of conflict resolution such as team-building activities that promote trust. As Pelled and Adler (1994) suggested, it is important to examine

the antecedents of conflict – specifically, the processes by which functional background heterogeneity induces conflict. ... . Although we focus on conflict inducing processes triggered by functional diversity, we expect that other kinds of diversity (gender, tenure, etc.) generate similar processes; however, we submit that these other kinds of diversity differ both in the degree to which they trigger these processes and in the contextual factors that moderate their effects. (p. 21)

Other authors have focused on people's responses to conflict. A popular model, based on extensive research in a variety of work groups (Blake & Mouton, 1964; De Dreu, Evers, Beersma, Kluwer, & Nauta, 2001; Wilmot & Hocker, 2001) has identified five typical responses: forcing, accommodating, avoiding, compromising, and problem solving. *Forcing* involves a person prioritizing his or her interests with the willingness to sacrifice the relationship with the other person to achieve those interests. By contrast, *accommodating* involves an individual sacrificing his or her own interests to diffuse the tension and preserve the relationship. An *avoiding* response involves a straightforward withdrawal from the conflict, so no resolution is attained. *Compromising* involves one or both parties giving up something to minimize the conflict. Finally, *problem solving* involves open communication about the disagreement and managing the conflict in a way that satisfies the interests of both parties. More recently, it has been recognized that individuals respond to conflict using a combination of styles, either sequentially or simultaneously (Munduate, Ganaza, Peiró, & Euwema, 1999; Van de Vliert, Euwema, & Husimans, 1995). In health care, it has been shown that providers tend to initially respond to conflict using an avoiding response, shift to forcing if the conflict continues, and resort to problem solving only as a last option (Skjørshammer, 2001). There are many models of conflict management and it is beyond the scope of this chapter to explore and compare them all. The point is that conflict is inevitable and, therefore, in addition to our educational efforts in teaching our learners to minimize conflict, it is important that we also provide learners with the ability to understand and manage conflict when it does arise.

DISCUSSION

Over the last decade, the concepts of effective IPC and IPE have become deeply entwined. It is largely taken for granted that IPE is the process by which we train collaborative practitioners. Yet there are likely assumptions built into our construction of IPC that, at best, translate poorly into our models of IPE. There are also likely assumptions built into our models of IPE that may, in fact, undermine the development of effective collaborative practices in the health care environment. In this chapter, we have offered an alternative model of IPC, one that is less focused on effective participation in collaborative teams and more focused on the development, nurturing, and sustaining of one's own effective collaborative networks. We suggest that such an approach may be valuable for participation in effectively collaborating teams, but does not require the presence of well-functioning collaborative teams to be useful and valuable as a model of IPC. Importantly, this model places the skills (and perhaps the responsibility) to develop collaborative relationships with other health care providers (and with the patient), in the hands of individual practitioners. In this sense, it puts the *"I"* in team.

As a step toward this reconstruction of training for IPC, we have offered four concepts (each of which likely would require further development as a set of knowledge, skills, and values) that an individual health care provider might profitably employ to develop, nurture, and sustain effective collaborations within and across professions and with patients and families: building social capital, perspective taking, negotiating priorities and resources, and managing conflict. Undoubtedly, if these concepts were understood and effectively enacted by all members of the health professional community, the collaborative process would be substantially smoother. However, what we find particularly intriguing about this model, is that those with whom one is interacting need not be particularly sophisticated in these concepts in order for the practices to be effective. In this sense, this approach opens the possibility of cracking the conundrum that we introduced in the introduction. That is, our current models have led us to teach skills of collaboration that require a collaborative environment to enact well. Thus, these models are trapped in a logical *cul-de-sac,* whereby we are attempting to change behaviors in order to shift the culture, but we must first change the culture for those behaviors to be effective. By contrast, the model proposed here has the potential to enable properly trained clinicians to individually be the change we want to see.

With these ideas in mind, we wish to return to the notion of training for collaboration and the assumptions built into the current construction of IPE at both pre- and post-licensure levels. We offer some insights into how preparation for effective collaboration might be viewed as we address training for collaboration in a non-collaborative world.

- We propose moving away from teaching how collaboration should work ideally and providing the skills to function if it did work that way, and moving instead toward teaching the reality of current practice and how one can nonetheless develop effective collaborative networks around oneself.
- We also suggest that these concepts be taught explicitly. Often current models of IPE involve placing different professionals together and setting forth tasks or conditions in which they must enact collaboration in order to accomplish the skills. The expectation is that by having to enact the skills, they will discover the skills spontaneously or develop the skills implicitly. We believe that theories of deliberate practice and reflective practice suggest that such skills are better used and developed when they are explicit.

- We note that IPE traditionally requires that all health care practitioners participate, yet all professions are rarely, if ever, fully engaged and invested in the IPE endeavor. By focusing IPC training on individual skills of developing collaborative networks, no one profession can undermine the effort. In fact, failure to participate might well put a profession at a disadvantage, as they would be less sophisticated in these concepts and, therefore, potentially at risk of being manipulated by them.

In practice, we offer a few examples of how we might enact the details of such a curriculum:

- As an example of a specific content area that might change, we might start thinking of not offering 'role clarification' (which implies rigid interfaces with others and possibly leads to stereotyping that is unprofitable in relationship building and negotiation). Rather, we might offer brief glimpses into how each profession generally constructs patient problems, what each tends to see as their daily challenges, and what tends to qualify as legitimate solutions. We could reinforce the tentative nature of these caricatures largely as a way of showing how perspectives can be different and provide the skills to explore each collaborator's answers to these questions in the particular situation on which one is collaborating.
- As an example of how we might address just one of the four domains, teaching perspective taking, may involve arranging for health care providers to explicitly practice actively considering the viewpoint of someone else. For example, we might begin by exposing learners to videos of conflict-laden interactions and training them to deliberately and repeatedly ask, while watching the interaction, "How might each person feel? What might each person be thinking?" This could be followed by reports from each of the actors in the encounter regarding how they actually did feel and what they actually did think. Such practices might then be extended to students' placements to decrease their tendency to interpret the complex interactions and activities they observe in the health care environment only through their own, relatively naïve, perspective. Eventually, the goal would be to teach them to consider the possibility of other perspectives when they are, themselves, embedded in the interaction.

CONCLUSION

Given the five or more decades since the idea that interprofessional health education could lead to collaborative, patient-centered practice was first identified, little has changed in its uptake until the last few years. With its growing traction, IPE has increasingly been taken for granted as a solution to IPC, and in many ways has created its own complex set of problems. Rather than trying to tackle these problems directly, we suggest thinking again about whether IPE as it is currently constructed is necessarily the solution. This leads us to re-examine the notion of effective IPC, and to the possibility that our intense focus on teams may have diverted us from another layer of collaboration that both focuses on the individual and acts as an antecedent to improved team work through earlier preparation of the individual team members: the building, nurturing, and sustaining of effective collaborative networks. Refocusing in this way raises the possibility that a different set of skills may be of particular relevance, and that different approaches to teaching these skills might be possible.

Of course, we do not intend this chapter to be the final word on these ideas. Undoubtedly there are other concepts that are important in thinking about network building, and we look forward to others adding reflectively to this list. We have at best touched only lightly on issues of institutional structures and the complexities of power relationships and how these factors might affect one's implementation of these concepts in a particular context or situation. As such, we intend this as the beginning of a conversation, as the skeleton of a framework to be modified, challenged, and elaborated.

REFERENCES

Adler, P. S., & Kwon, S.-W. (2002). Social capital: Prospects for a new concept. *Academy of Management Review, 27,* 17–40.

Appelbaum, S. H., Abdallah, C., & Shapiro, B. T. (1999). The self-directed team: A conflict resolution analysis. *Team Performance Management, 5*(2), 60–77. http://dx.doi.org/10.1108/13527599910268940.

Baker, G. R., Norton, P. G., Flintoft, V., Blais, R., Brown, A., Cox, J., . . . Tamblyn, R. (2004). The Canadian adverse events study: The incidence of adverse events among hospital patients in Canada. *CMAJ, 170,* 1678–1686. http://dx.doi.org/10.1503/cmaj.1040498.

Bakhtin, M. M. (1981). The dialogic imagination: Four essays by MM Bakhtin (C. Emerson & M. Holquist, Trans.). Austin, TX: University of Texas Press.

Batson, C. D. (1991). The altruism question: Toward a social-psychological answer. Hillsdale, NJ: Erlbaum.

Blake, R. R., & Mouton, J. S. (1964). The managerial grid. Houston, TX: Gulf.

Boland, R. J., Jr., & Tenkasi, R. V. (1995). Perspective Making and perspective taking in communities of knowing. *Organization Science, 6*(4), 350–372. http://dx.doi.org/10.1287/orsc.6.4.350.

Bolden, R., & Gosling, J. (2006). Leadership competencies: Time to change the tune? Leadership 2, 147–163. http://dx.doi.org/10.1177/1742715006062932.

Bourdieu, P. (1986). The forms of capital. In J. Richardson (Ed.), Handbook of theory and research for the sociology of education (pp. 241–258). New York, NY: Greenwood.

Brown, R. (1981). Social psychology. New York, NY: The Free Press.

Canadian Interprofessional Health Collaborative. (2010). A national interprofessional competency framework. Retrieved from http://www.cihc.ca/files/CIHC_IP Competencies_Feb1210.pdf.

Centre for the Advancement of Interprofessional Education. (2002). Defining IPE. Retrieved from http://caipe.org.uk/about-us/defining-ipe/.

Cialdini, R. B., Brown, S. L., Lewis, B. P., Luce, C., & Neuberg, S. L. (1997). Reinterpreting the empathy – altruism relationship: When one into one equals oneness. *Journal of Personality and Social Psychology, 73,* 481–494. http://dx.doi.org/10.1037//0022-3514.73.3.481.

Coleman, J. S. (1988). Social capital in the creation of human capital. *American Journal of Sociology, 94*(Suppl.), S95–S120.

Davis, M. H., Conklin, L., Smith, A., & Luce, C. (1996). Effect of perspective taking on the cognitive representation of persons: A merging of self and other. *Journal of Personality and Social Psychology, 70,* 713–726. http://dx.doi.org/10.1037//0022-3514.70.4.713.

De Dreu, C. K. W., Evers, A., Beersma, B., Kluwer, E. S., & Nauta, A. (2001). A theory-based measure of conflict management strategies in the workplace. *Journal of Organizational Behavior, 22,* 645–668. http://dx.doi.org/10.1002/job.107.

De Dreu, C. K. W., & Weingart, L. R. (2003). Task versus relationship conflict, team performance, and team member satisfaction: A meta-analysis. *Journal of Applied Psychology, 88,* 741–749. http://dx.doi.org/10.1037/0021-9010.88.4.741.

Deutsch, M. (1994). Constructive conflict resolution: Principles, training and research. *Journal of Social Issues, 50,* 13–32. http://dx.doi.org/10.1111/j.1540-4560.1994. tb02395.x.

Epley, N., Keysar, B., Van Boven, L., & Gilovich, T. (2004). Perspective taking as egocentric anchoring and adjustment. *Journal of Personality and Social Psychology, 87,* 327–339. http://dx.doi.org/10.1037/0022-3514.87.3.327

Frenk, J., Chen, L., Bhutta, Z. A., Cohen, J., Crisp, N., Evans, T., . . . Zurayk, H. (2010). Health professionals for a new century:Transforming education to strengthen health systems in an interdependent world. *The Lancet, 376,* 1923–1958. http://dx.doi.org/10.1016/S0140-6736(10)61854-5.

Galinsky, A. D., & Moskowitz, G. B. (2000). Perspective-taking: Decreasing stereotype expression, stereotype accessibility, and in-group favoritism. *Journal of Personality and Social Psychology, 78,* 708–724. http://dx.doi.org/10.1037/0022-3514.78.4.708.

Galinsky, A. D., & Moskowitz, G. B. (2001). First offers as anchors: The role of perspective-taking and negotiator focus. *Journal of Personality and Social Psychology, 81,* 657–669. http://dx.doi.org/10.1037/0022-3514.81.4.657/

Gofton, W., & Regehr, G. (2006). What we don't know we are teaching: Unveiling the hidden curriculum. *Clinical Orthopaedics and Related Research,* 449, 20–27. http://dx.doi.org/10.1097/01.blo.0000224024.96034.b2.

Goldman, J., Meuser, J., Rogers, J., Lawrie, L., & Reeves, S. (2010). Interprofessional collaboration in family health teams: An Ontario-based study. *Canadian Family Physician,* 56(10), e368–e374.

Hafferty, F. W. (1998). Beyond curriculum reform: Confronting medicine's hidden curriculum. *Academic Medicine, 73,* 403–407.

Holmes, C. L., Harris, I. B., Schwartz, A. J., & Regehr, G. (2014). Harnessing the hidden curriculum: A four-step approach to developing and reinforcing reflective competencies in medical clinical clerkship. Advances in Health Science Education: Theory and Practice, Advance online publication. http://dx.doi.org/10.1007/s10459-014-9558-9.

Jehn, K. A. (1994). Enhancing effectiveness: An investigation of advantages and disadvantages of value-based intragroup conflict. *International Journal of Conflict Management,* 5, 223–238. http://dx.doi.org/10.1108/eb022744.

Krauss, R. M., & Fussell, S. R. (1991). Perspective-taking in communication: Representations of others' knowledge in reference. *Social Cognition,* 9(1), 2–24.

Leung, A., Luu, S., Regehr, G., Murnaghan, M. L., Gallinger, S., & Moulton, C. A. (2012). "First, do no harm": Balancing competing priorities in surgical practice. *Academic Medicine,* 87, 1368–1374.

Lingard, L., Espin, S., Evans, C., & Hawryluck, L. (2004). The rules of the game: Interprofessional collaboration on the intensive care unit team. *Critical Care,* 8(6), R403–R408. http://dx.doi.org/10.1186/cc2958.

Lingard, L., Garwood, S., & Poenaru, D. (2004). Tensions influencing operating room team function: Does institutional context make a difference? *Medical Education,* 38, 691–699.

Manning, T., & Robertson, B. (2003a). Influencing and negotiating skills: Some research and reflections, part I: Influencing strategies and styles. *Industrial and Commercial Training* 35, 11–15. http://dx.doi.org/10.1108/00197850310458180.

Manning, T., & Robertson, B. (2003b). Influencing and negotiating skills: Some research and reflections, part II: Influencing styles and negotiating skills. *Industrial and Commercial Training,* 35, 60–66. http://dx.doi.org/10.1108/00197850310463760.

Manning, T., & Robertson, B. (2004). Influencing, negotiating skills and conflict-handling: Some additional research and reflections. *Industrial and Commercial Training,* 36, 104–109. http://dx.doi.org/10.1108/00197850410532104.

Munduate, L., Ganaza, J., Peiró, J. M., & Euwema, M. (1999). Patterns of styles in conflict management and effectiveness. *International Journal of Conflict Management,* 10, 5–24. http://dx.doi.org/10.1108/eb022816.

Pelled, L. H., & Adler, P. S. (1994). Antecedents of intergroup conflict in multifunctional product development teams: A conceptual model. *IEEE Transactions on Engineering Management,* 41(1), 21–28.

Prescott, P. A., & Bowen, S. A. (1985). Physician–nurse relationships. *Annals of Internal Medicine,* 103, 127–133. http://dx.doi.org/10.7326/0003-4819-103-1-127.

Putnam, R. D. (1993). The prosperous community: Social capital and public life. *The American Prospect,* 13, 35–42.

Putnam, R. D. (1995). Bowling alone: American's declining social capital. *Journal of Democracy,* 6(1), 65–78.

Rogers, D. A., & Lingard, L. (2006). Surgeons managing conflict: A framework for understanding the challenge. *Journal of the American College of Surgeons,* 203, 568–574. http://dx.doi.org/10.1016/j.jamcollsurg.2006.06.012.

Schulz, K. (2010). Being wrong: Adventures in the margin of error. New York, NY: Harper Collins.

Simons, T. L., & Peterson, R. S. (2000). Task conflict and relationship conflict in top management teams: The pivotal role of intragroup trust. *Journal of Applied Psychology,* 85(1), 102–111. http://dx.doi.org/10.1037//0021-9010.85.1.102.

Skjørshammer, M. (2001). Co-operation and conflict in a hospital: Interprofessional differences in perception and management of conflicts. *Journal of Interprofessional Care,* 15, 7–18. http://dx.doi.org/10.1080/13561820020022837.

Studdert, D. M., Burns, J. P., Mello, M. M., Puopolo, A. L., Truog, R. D., & Brennan, T. A. (2003). Nature of conflict in the care of pediatric intensive care patients with prolonged stay. *Pediatrics,* 112(3 Pt 1), 553–558. http://dx.doi.org/10.1542/peds.112.3.553.

Studdert, D. M., Mello, M. M., Burns, J. P., Puopolo, A. L., Galper, B. Z., Truog, R. D., & Brennan, T. A. (2003). Conflict in the care of patients with prolonged stay in the ICU:

Types, sources, and predictors. Intensive Care Medicine, 29, 1489–1497. http://dx.doi.org/10.1007/s00134-003-1853-5.

Suter, E., & Deutschlander, S. (2010). Can interprofessional collaboration provide health human resources solutions? A knowledge synthesis. Retrieved from http://www.cihc.ca/files/FinalSynthesisReportMarch2010. pdf.

Szaz, G. (1968). Second interim report of the committee on interprofessional education in the health sciences. Vancouver, Canada: Health Sciences Centre, University of British Columbia.

Thomas, K. W. (1992). Conflict and conflict management: Reflections and update. *Journal of Organizational Behavior,* 13, 265–274. http://dx.doi.org/10.1002/job.4030130307.

Van de Vliert, E., Euwema, M. C., Husimans, S. E. (1995). Managing conflict with a subordinate or a superior: Effectiveness of conglomerated behavior. *Journal of Applied Psychology,* 80, 271–281. http://dx.doi.org/10.1037/0021-9010.80.2.271.

Way, D., Jones, L., & Busing, N. (2000). Implementation strategies: "Collaboration in primary care –family doctors & nurse practitioners delivering shared care" [Discussion paper]. Retrieved from http://www.eicp.ca/en/toolkit/management-leadership/ocfp-paper-handout.pdf.

Wilmot, W. W., & Hocker, J. L. (2001). Interpersonal conflict (6th ed.). Boston, MA: McGraw-Hill.

World Health Organization. (2010). Framework for action on interprofessional education & collaborative practice. Retrieved from http://whqlibdoc.who.int/hq/2010/WHO_HRH_HPN_10.3_eng.pdf?ua=1.

In: Interprofessional Client-Centred Collaborative Practice   ISBN: 978-1-63483-754-5
Editor: Carole Orchard   © 2015 Nova Science Publishers, Inc.

Chapter 5

CHANGING ORGANIZATIONAL CULTURE TO EMBRACE INTERPROFESSIONAL EDUCATION AND INTERPROFESSIONAL PRACTICE

Ivy Oandasan

Department of Family and Community Medicine,
University of Toronto, Toronto, ON, Canada

ABSTRACT

Advancing interprofessional education (IPE) and interprofessional practice (IPC) requires a cultural shift that is supported and led by all those who are part of the healthcare system. This chapter shares the story of how one province in Canada was able to mobilize a movement of change using learning opportunities that stimulated reflection in order to create transformative action. Using educational and organizational development literature, the chapter highlights theories used to create cultural shifts within organizations, with the people who work within them, and across the healthcare system. By the end of the chapter, readers will see how theory can be put into action, engaging hundreds to create the cultural shift needed to enable interprofessional client-centered care.

Keywords: Organizational culture, interprofessional practice, system change, transformative change, reflection, change, culture shift, systems level, advocacy

INTRODUCTION

Worldwide, there has been a movement calling for a change in the way we deliver healthcare using a health workforce that works collaboratively to enhance access and improved client outcomes (World Health Organization 2010). The desire to be more client centered, empowering clients to be partners in their care and valuing their voices, is being advocated strongly (College of Family Physicians of Canada. A vision for Canada. Family practice: the patient's medical home. Mississauga, ON: College of Family Physicians of Canada; 2011. Available from: www.cfpc.ca/uploadedFiles/Resources/Resource Items/ PMH_A_Vision_for_Canada.pdf. 2011; Davis, Schoen and Schoenbaum 2000; Institute of Medicine 2001). Leaders from across the healthcare and health professions education systems are influencing cultural shifts. They are enabling new approaches, demonstrating that collaborative client-centered care improves not only client outcomes but also health care provider satisfaction and better system efficiencies. The cultural norms developed by people are now being changed by people. But how? How can we change the culture of what has been, to what we collectively want?

This chapter will review concepts that highlight the role of reflection in enabling transformative change. Individuals collectively make up organizations, and organizations collectively make up systems. It is through the actions of individuals that change happens. This chapter provides examples of how one province in Canada was able to catalyze a movement of reflection to enable action. Individuals from across the healthcare system were invited to enter into a dialogue, and through their voices, language was found to describe the types of changes needed to advance a culture to support quality-focused, collaborative, client-centered care.

It is rare for healthcare organizations and the individuals within them to take the time to reflect upon what can be done at a systems level to enhance healthcare delivery. The dearth of collaboration among organizations resembles the lack of collaboration that often exists among healthcare providers. The type of strategies needed to advance collaboration between healthcare education and health professional organizations resembles the type of strategies needed to advance interprofessional care with healthcare providers. The common denominator lies in the individuals who are part of the healthcare system, those who provide, support, and enable the delivery of care for clients. Change needed within the healthcare system requires the majority of individuals who are part of the system to uncover for themselves those changes that need to happen. Through their reflections, decisions are made that either stimulate or preempt action. Change is only possible if individuals see the need for change.

INTERPROFESSIONAL EDUCATION AS A FORM OF ADVOCACY

The magnitude of change that we, as leaders advancing IPE and interprofessional client-centered care, see is a revolutionary one. International reports including the World Health Organization's (2010) *Framework for Action on Interprofessional Education and Collaborative Practice* have recognized the need for systems change. According to the World Health Organization report, educators, practitioners, policymakers, leaders, government, students, and clients and their families all have a part to play. The fundamental premise of IPE is to enable health care professionals to collaborate to provide quality, focused, client-centered care. As educators, our role is more tangibly seen with our learners. Yet, as IPE educators, we have an extended role, that of advocating for patients or clients who are often voiceless, powerless, and lost in the complexity of the healthcare system. As interprofessional educationalists, we advocate for systems change. Oandasan and Barker (2005) provided the following description of health advocacy:

Purposeful actions by health professionals to address determinants of health which negatively impact individuals or communities by either informing those who can enact change or by initiating, mobilizing, and organizing activities to make change happen, with or on behalf of the individuals or communities with whom health professionals work. (p. S41)

Oandasan and Barker's (2005) definition, derived from Ezell (2001), suggests that advocacy is a practice or an action. It is more than a set of thoughts, feelings, or attitudes. Ezell further emphasized that advocacy "consists of purposive efforts to change specific existing or proposed policies or practices on behalf of or with a specific client or group of clients" (p. 23). To this end, individuals undertaking advocacy work are involved in deliberate and purposeful efforts to support change. As leaders involved in IPE, we rarely see our work as a form of advocacy but could we, and should we?

USING EDUCATIONAL THEORIES TO FOSTER CHANGE

Paolo Friere (2002) in his book *Pedagogy of the Oppressed* believed that education is a form of activism (p. 51). He believed that when *praxis* (or reflection) and *action* are enabled, transformation is possible. Transformative learning, coined by Mezirow (1991) describes the process of learning that involves "using a prior interpretation to construe a new or revised interpretation of the meaning of one's experience in order to guide future action" (p. 12). Both Friere and Mezirow link the process of internal individual reflection with external opportunities for action. The internal reflection experienced by an individual often leads to a deep shift in perspective, resulting in noticeable changes in action due to the shift (Cranton 2011). This shift, also described as a perspective transformation (Mezirow 1991) implies that when an individual critically reflects, he or she becomes aware of his or her own frames of reference or perceptions. In the IPE literature, the act of reflection is often cited as a skill needed by health care providers to successfully implement IPC (Clark 2009; D'Eon 2005; Oandasan and Reeves, 2005). Reflection occurs at multiple levels, for example with one's self, while being with others, and in different contexts. Schön's (1991) concept of there reflective practitioner aligns well with what we expect of competent interprofessional collaborators. As described by Schön, reflective practitioners are able to use reflection to learn from and to frame forward ways to address complex and murky problems faced in professional practice. Used in the practice of interprofessional care, reflecting on one's actions and the actions of others can help facilitate (a) *who* to call upon when needing to collaborate, (b) *how* to communicate effectively to facilitate care plans, and (c) *what* to do when differences of opinion arise. These competencies are highlighted in many of the competency frameworks published related to IPE and IPC (Brewer and Jones 2013; Canadian Interprofessional Health Collaborative, 2010; Interprofessional Education Collaborative Expert Panel 2011). Fundamental to all of the IPE and IPC competencies is the ability to reflect. Mann, Gordon, and MacLeod (2009) recognized that researchers using reflection and reflective practice as primary interventions in their inquiries have found it challenging to document definitive impact. Mann et al.'s systematic literature review noted that despite the lack of definitive evidence, reflective interventions, when used in learning situations, can influence individual perceptions, which in turn can affect client care outcomes. It is the transfer or application of new perspectives that IPC advocates hope will continue to catalyze the IPE movement in support of the delivery of interprofessional care. What healthcare providers often forget is that the opportunities to learn continue well beyond the four walls of the academic ivory towers of colleges and universities from which they graduated. By recognizing that clinical settings provide ideal opportunities to engage in day-to-day learning, those of us trying to advance interprofessional ways of practice have a new context to play within—the real day-to-day life found in practice settings.

The opportunity to provide continuing IPE within practice organizations, supporting staff to learn about, from, and with three or more healthcare providers to advance collaboration and improved client outcomes (World Health Organization 2010) is ripe for the taking. It is through this learning that transformative possibilities for advancing IPE and IPC can happen.

CREATING A LEARNING CULTURE TO ADVANCE INTERPROFESSIONAL CLIENT-CENTERED CARE

While all individuals have the capacity to learn, Senge (2006) asserts that organizations have not capitalized on opportunities to offer reflection and engagement opportunities to support continued learning. Senge brought forward the idea of creating learning organizations, which he described as

> organizations where people continually expand their capacity to create the results they truly desire, where new and expansive patterns of thinking are nurtured, where collective aspiration is set free, and where people are continually learning to see the whole together (p. 4).

According to Senge (2006), learning organizations are structured to enable individuals within them to build a shared vision, test their individual and collective mental models, support personal mastery, implement team learning, and advocate for systems thinking.

These five disciplines, Senge argues, should be embedded within the fabric of any organization that strives to excel. The culture of an organization is comprised of widely shared and deeply held values, beliefs, and assumptions of the people within it (Schein 1993). If Senge's five disciplines are believed as fundamental to what individuals within an organization should do, then these actions must be carried out willingly by the majority before it becomes a norm within an organization. Culture, according to Schein (1993), is shaped by the underlying beliefs and assumptions of individuals guiding what they do.

These beliefs and assumptions are derived from day-to-day problem solving that works well enough for individuals to consider that the approaches are valid and appropriate. Thus, these approaches are taught to new members as they become part of an organization and become the correct way to perceive, think, and feel when faced with similar problems. If, therefore, interprofessional care becomes considered the best approach to provide care to clients, then over time this approach will be taught to new individuals and shared across all who work within an organization.

While this is the hope, enabling interprofessional care to become the norm requires individuals to believe that it is the fundamental approach to practice guiding all that they do. Helping individuals shift their old mental models to new ones is possible within learning organizations. To change a system, the mental models must be shifted across those involved in healthcare.

EMBRACING ALL PARTS OF THE WHOLE IN ADVANCING IPE AND IPC

As noted in D'Amour and Oandasan's (2005) evolving framework for advancing interprofessional education for collaborative patient-centered practice (IECPCP; see Figure IV), two major systems — the education system and the professional system — act interdependently to enable both IPE and IPC to be implemented.

Each system consists of linkages within and across systems, reflecting the determinants and processes of collaboration required at several levels, including links among learners, teachers, and professionals (i.e., the micro level); links at the organizational level between teaching and health organizations (i.e., the meso level); and links among systems such as the political, socio-economic, regulatory, and cultural systems (i.e., macro level).

In each system and at each level, thousands of individuals exist. System change, therefore, requires individuals in each system and at each level to commit to change. The multiplicity of individuals involved in advancing IPE and IPC is staggering, begging the question if it can be done.

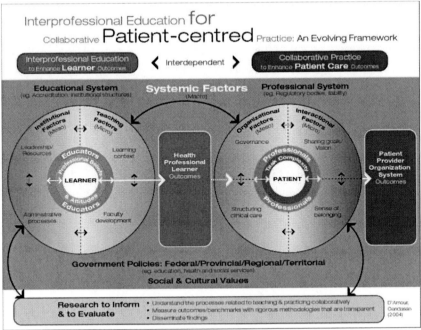

Note. From "Interprofessionality as the Field of Interprofessional Practice and Interprofessional Education: An Emerging Concept," by D. D'Amour and I. Oandasan, 2005, *Journal of Interprofessional Care, 19*(Suppl. 1), p. 11. Copyright 2005 by D'Amour and Oandasan. Reprinted with permission.

Figure IV. Interprofessional education for collaborative patient-centered practice model.

THE STORY OF ADVANCING INTERPROFESSIONAL CLIENT-CENTERED CARE IN THE PROVINCE OF ONTARIO

What if it was possible to enable organizations and the leaders who work within them to dialog and learn, about, from and with each other in order to find ways to collaborate to improve the delivery of care within the healthcare system? How might this story be told? What follows, is a short story describing how one province in Canada facilitated a process to enable healthcare system leaders to engage in dialog, enabling them to reflect and uncover a shared vision for the type of health care they want to collectively provide the citizens of their province. This shared vision, founded upon similar values, beliefs, and assumptions, helped to catalyze the movement for IPE and IPC in this province.

The story began in 2005, when leaders across Canada were advocating for the advancement of IECPCP (D'Amour and Oandasan 2005) through an initiative funded by Health Canada. Herbert (2005) highlighted details of this national movement. With the release of the IECPCP framework (Figure IV), it was recognized that the successful adoption of IPE and IPC rested upon the engagement and involvement of stakeholder across the healthcare system.

Spurred on by D'Amour and Oandasan's (2005) IECPCP framework, the opportunity to bring the framework to life in one province emerged. In 2005, the Assistant Deputy Minister of Health who had the portfolio of Health Human Resources was Dr. Joshua Tepper. He believed the province needed more than just additional health professionals. He said, "I knew we had to do things differently" (Tepper, as cited in Nelson, Tassone, and Hodges 2014, p. 20). A group of IPE and IPC advocates arranged a meeting with Dr. Tepper (a recently graduated family physician new to the Assistant Deputy Minister of Health role) with a goal of seeking his support to test Ontario's readiness to advance IPE and IPC in the province. The outcome of the 1-hour meeting, which took place in the early part of 2005, was an agreement by government to fund an invitational summit to be held in June of 2005, with 100 leaders representing the education, practice, regulation, government, accreditation, research, and health professional association sectors of the healthcare system. The leaders who participated in the 1-day event unanimously believed in the importance of interprofessional care and called for action (Interprofessional Care Advisory Group 2006).

The invitational summit agenda was loosely designed using an appreciative inquiry (AI) approach (Cooperrider and Whitney 1999). AI is used in organizational development to help individuals think in more positive and generative ways enabling transformational change (Marshak and Grant 2008). AI engages individuals to reflect upon and share stories of what is currently working so as to help them collectively discover relevant and meaningful ways to approach change. By being part of conversations, identifying relevant solutions, and motivating oneself and peers to act, transformational shifts are made possible (Bushe and Kassam 2005).

Designed with a combination of speakers and interactive table discussions, the summit engaged participants in multiple opportunities to share stories and perspectives and challenge opinions and beliefs. The leaders in attendance were assigned seating to ensure there was a mix of perspectives from all parts of the healthcare system and representation from across regions. One of the highlights of the summit was the story told by Carole Laurin (as cited in Oandasan 2006), a woman who had suffered a stroke and experienced failures among healthcare providers to hear her voice, needs, and hopes (client-centered care). In her story, Carole (as cited in Oandasan 2006) shared her conviction that the health care system needs to support the delivery of interprofessional care through seamless services for people such as herself, whose care trajectory touches hundreds of health care providers, is offered within dozens of healthcare organizations, and is influenced by many of the leaders and policy and decision makers at all levels of the education and health professional systems who were in attendance in the room. The intentional use of her narrative was aimed to create a reflective opportunity, stimulating those in the room to consider their mental models of their organizations' roles and abilities to deliver healthcare to clients with others as part of a system. Successful transformative learning opportunities inspire action, especially when individuals are faced with uncomfortable truths, values, and beliefs that are discordant with their own intentions. As Cranton (2011) suggests, learning is not transformative unless a person, group, or larger social unit encounters a perspective that is at odds with a prevailing perspective and a deep shift occurs with noticeable changes in actions as a result of the shift. The design of the summit set aside time for reflection using purposeful questions to incite dialog. Leaders in the room, used the client narrative, and presentations about the evidence related to IPE and IPC to consider the challenges, opportunities and priorities needed to individually and collectively advance IPE and IPC in the province. The end result of the invitational summit was a description of a healthcare system that enabled individuals, organizations, and all parts of the system to work together to identify actions in order to create the transformational change of realigning the system to be more centered around clients' needs and hopes. A vision for the future state of the healthcare system was shared with a description of what healthcare providers, healthcare organizations, and broader health system stakeholders need to do to support IPE and IPC (Figure V). As a sign of their commitment, all stakeholders in the room signed the Invitational Summit Poster (see Figure VI) to symbolically commemorate the collective vision and commitment created that day to advance IPC and IPE in the province of Ontario. Tepper (as cited in Nelson et al. 2014) reported that he received the support needed to push the IPE–IPC and quality care agenda for Ontario from the voices of leaders, many of whom were in the room that day (p. 21). The idea to create an Interprofessional Care Blueprint for Action was launched and heartily supported.

Led by Tom Closson, a well-known healthcare leader in Ontario, and Ivy Oandasan, the co-author of the IECPCP framework (D'Amour and Oandasan 2005), the two co-chairs were named to facilitate the process of creating the IPC Blueprint for Action with support from government.

A steering committee of Ontario experts in the fields of policy, education, regulation, and organizational structure was struck in the fall of 2006. Leveraging again the AI approach (Cooperrider and Whitney 1999), the development of the blueprint used similar techniques to bring influential leaders across the health care system into dialog, engage them in opportunities of reflection, and support processes to help co-create actions to catalyze transformational change. Three working groups were struck to support advancements needed to implement IPE and IPC across the Province of Ontario: organizational infrastructure, education, and regulation. Each working group included individuals who were considered influential in sectors that include hospitals, community health agencies, colleges, universities, regulatory bodies, accreditors, professional associations, insurance agencies, and unions.

5.1   A Common Vision for Interprofessional Care

The following concepts were common to all the small groups as they discussed an overall vision of interprofessional care.

What it looks like:

- A safe, effective, and seamless continuum of care designed for each individual, where plans are created and in which roles are clearly defined and delivery of care is patient-centred.

All health care providers

- must have a clear and thorough understanding of the competencies of the other health care professionals. Mutual respect for roles and skills set must be present among health care professionals. Clarity about each professional's role is important.
- must have an understanding of the patient populations that do best within the interprofessional care model. Interprofessional care may not be necessary, or desirable, in all cases. Research is needed to clearly identify who would do well and who would do poorly in different kinds of health care settings.

Health care organizations and institutions

- must have a common vision of and language for what "health" means as it relates to interprofessional care, and
- should have interprofessional care as part of a comprehensive strategy (individual, team, institution). Policies should acknowledge that teaching and practice are inter-related.

The health care system and its stakeholders:

- must be committed to change.
- must be prepared for cultural shift to get to team-based, balanced, equitable collaboration for patient-centred care.
- will change only if there is dynamic leadership, competent practitioners, and financial support.
- will need interprofessional care as the cornerstone for its province-wide health human resource strategy.

Note. From Proceedings Report for the Summit on Advancing Interprofessional Education and Practice(p. 26), by Ontario Ministry of Health and Long-Term Care in partnership with the Office of Interprofessional Education at the University of Toronto and the Ontario Ministry of Training, Colleges and Universities, 2006, Ottawa, ON, Canada: Queen's Printer. Copyright by Ontario Ministry of Health and Long-Term Care in partnership with the Office of Interprofessional Education at the University of Toronto and the Ontario Ministry of Training, Colleges and Universities, 2006, Proceedings Report for the Summit on Advancing Interprofessional Education and Practice pg. 26. Reprinted with permission.

Figure V. A common vision for interprofessional care, IPC Summit, June 2006.

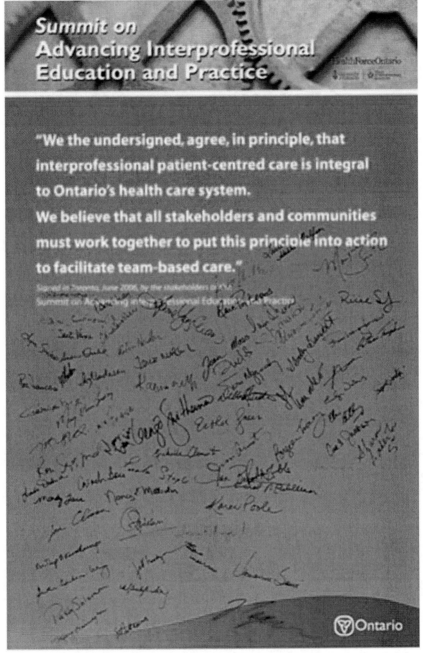

Note. From Proceedings Report for the Summit on Advancing Interprofessional Education and
     Practice(p. 3), by Ontario Ministry of Health and Long-Term Care in partnership with the Office of
     Interprofessional Education at the University of Toronto and the Ontario Ministry of Training,
     Colleges and Universities, 2006, Ottawa, ON, Canada: Queen's Printer. Copyright by Ontario
     Ministry of Health and Long-Term Care in partnership with the Office of Interprofessional
     Education at the University of Toronto and the Ontario Ministry of Training, Colleges and
     Universities, 2006, PROCEEDINGS REPORT for the Summit on Advancing Interprofessional
     Education and Practice pg. 3. Reprinted with permission.

Figure VI. Commitment of support for IPE and IPC, 2006.

The working groups were charged with creating recommendations for actions to advance IPC while still aligning with the province's health system strategic directions that included enhancing wait times and improving chronic disease management (Interprofessional Care Steering Committee [IPCSC], 2007).

The three groups developed short-term, intermediate, and long-term action-oriented activities to facilitate IPC at all levels (micro, meso, and macro). Each activity articulated individual, shared, and collective roles of the different players and parts of the health care system. Just prior to the release of the blueprint, a further stakeholder consultation session was held at which the four major themes highlighted in the document were presented for validation:

1. "Create a firm foundation upon which key interprofessional activities can be built and sustained" (IPCSC 2007, p. 10).
2. "Share the responsibility for making sure interprofessional strategies are effectively implemented among [stakeholders]" (IPCSC 2007, p. 10).
3. Implement "systemic enablers" (IPCSC 2007, p. 10) that "allow interprofessional care to be taught, practiced and organized in a systemic way" (p. 10).
4. "Lead [a] sustainable cultural change that recognizes the . . . [transformative] nature of interprofessional care and embraces it at all levels" (IPCSC 2007, p. 10) of an organization.

For this process, participants who had attended the original invitational summit and others considered influential in advancing actions identified in the blueprint (IPCSC, 2007) were asked to provide feedback and hence inviting engagement. The blueprint was widely released in July of 2007 (IPCSC 2007), one year after the invitational summit. The result of this collaborative and consultative process left people feeling they had had a significant role in the blueprint's creation and a sense of ownership.

Earlier in the chapter the description of Senge's (2006) learning organizations was shared, identifying five interwoven forces or disciplines that need to be implemented for success: build a shared vision, test individual and collective mental models, support personal mastery, implement team learning, and advocate for systems thinking. The healthcare system is not one organization structured within four physical walls. However, if we were to imagine placing invisible walls around all of its parts, thinking of the healthcare system as a virtual organization, the diagram might look similar to that of D'Amour and Oandasan's (2005) IECPCP framework presented in Figure IV. The invitational summit and the work done after to develop the Blueprint for Action (IPCSC, 2007) created opportunities for healthcare leaders to reflect on their individual and collective roles within this virtual organization as members of one large healthcare team.

All who participated reflected upon their own values, beliefs, and assumptions to test and sharpen their mental models and to uncover and co-create new perspectives. Collectively, a shared vision of a better healthcare system was imagined, built upon the best of what each part could contribute (personal mastery). The leaders, together, engaged in team learning and systems thinking. Transformational learning requires that stakeholders reflect, interpret, challenge, reinterpret, and review, which enhances organizational performance and work outcomes, especially if learning occurs in teams (Choy 2009). Putting system leaders together through transformational learning opportunities founded upon dialog enables members of a system to challenge and reflect upon individual and collective actions, supporting new ways of thinking, and enabling opportunities for innovation to support continue improvement. By creating interprofessional opportunities that involved reflection, a shared vision and a shared action plan for interprofessional care was made possible in the Province of Ontario.

EVIDENCE OF CHANGE

Further work was subsequently carried out to implement the IPC Blueprint for Action in December 2007 (IPCSC 2007). The Interprofessional Care Strategic Implementation Committee (2010) was struck, charged to disseminate and implement actions described in the IPC Blueprint for Action (IPCSC 2007).Changes began to be seen, manifesting across different parts of the healthcare system (Interprofessional Care Strategic Implementation Committee 2010). A decade later, the vision of IPC and IPE continues to be seen, with more and more individuals engaged and committed to do their part in advancing IPE and IPC. Although there has not been a published evaluation of the IPC Blueprint for Action (IPCSC 2007) and its impact on the system, a number of key changes are shared as anecdotal evidence of shifts supporting the value of providing interprofessional care in the system aligned with structure, practice, policy, and behavioral changes.

1. Education and government sectors advancement of structural changes. To advance IPC, the Blueprint (IPCSC 2007) advocated for seamless integration between the education system that prepares the health workforce and the practice system, which employs and deploys its graduates. As part of Tepper's Assistant Deputy Minister of Health role to facilitate two parts of government, the Government of Ontario Ministry of Health and Long-Term Care and the Ministry of Training, Colleges, and Universities provided joint annual funding to support six Ontario Academic Health Science Centers (AHSCs) to purposively promote the development, implementation, and ongoing evaluation of core interprofessional education curricula for their health professional students. Each of the AHSCs were asked to include other universities and local colleges with health science programs in their individual initiatives to foster collaborative opportunities across the province (Interprofessional Care Strategic Implementation Committee, 2010). To this day, these institutions have maintained a structure within their AHSCs through either hiring a lead or creating offices or centers to help coordinate the development and implementation of IPE. Many, like the University of Toronto, have permanently created requisite curricula for all their health professional students who undertake training at the institution (Nelson et al. 2014).

2. Advancing behavioral and leadership changes in practice settings. To enable the practice of IPC, the "Advancing the Competence in Interprofessional Care: Charter on Expectation and Commitments" (Oandasan et al. 2009, p. 2) framework was developed. The charter, created by multiple stakeholders and built upon the narratives of patients and healthcare providers, described what interprofessional care is like at its best. The charter sets out a common language for what is expected by clients in relation to their interprofessional care and what healthcare providers and leaders can do to support IPC. The framework provides a descriptive model for successful IPC behaviors and attitudes. The language used aligns with already existing competency frameworks employed by academia across Canada, including the Canadian Interprofessional Health Collaborative (2010) IP

Collaboration competency framework. The advantage of the charter was the intuitive language and reflection tools used for healthcare providers, which when applied could perhaps influence change. Beyond the framework, other models of care also emerged in Ontario, including the creation of 150 family health teams to advance team-based care in primary care (Meuser, Bean, Goldman and Reeves 2006). Leadership positions also began to emerge with interprofessional portfolios (e.g., Vice President Interprofessional Education and Interprofessional Practice Leaders and Directors across numerous hospitals in the province). Thus, the use of the term *interprofessional* became more pervasive throughout the Ontario health system.

3. *Regulatory and government policy changes.* The Health Professions Regulatory Advisory Council (2009), an advisory group to Ontario's Minister of Health and Long-Term Care, recommended that the Regulated Health Professions Act (1991) needed to be updated to reflect the new reality of interprofessional care. The Health Professions Regulatory Advisory Council believed that professional regulatory bodies could not effectively ensure the competency of its professionals if they did not address members' readiness to work interprofessionally and their accountability to work as members of interprofessional care teams. In response, Ontario made IPC one of the statutory objectives of all regulatory bodies and implemented scope of practice changes across the regulated health professions in 2009 (Interprofessional Care Strategic Implementation Committee 2010). As Coffey and Anyinam (2015) noted, Ontario "clearly ended the neutrality of its health professional legislation on the responsibility of self-regulation to contribute to interprofessional collaboration" (p. 199).

Tosti and Jackson (1994) assert that congruence between the values of an organization and the values of the people within the organization is demonstrated when an organization's strategic goals and values support its objectives, are enacted through appropriate management practices, and align with people's activities. Earlier in the chapter we began discussing the concept of culture and how some assert that an organization's culture is embedded in artifacts that can be seen (Schein 1993). Culture, then, can be tangibly described through examining language used, organizational structures created, leadership models implemented, policies enacted and practices employed. If we can see the healthcare system as a learning organization, with all its different sectors as part of a whole, then maybe cultural shifts are possible and these shifts can be seen.

CONCLUSION

This chapter laid out the premise that change occurs through individuals taking actions guided by their personal and professional underlying values, beliefs, and assumptions. Their actions help to shape an organization's or system's culture. Given the worldwide movement to foster interprofessional client-centered approaches to care, strategies are needed to help stimulate change. Advancing interprofessional client-centered care necessitates a re-alignment of the healthcare system, with particular attention paid to the structures, policies, practices, and behaviors of organizations and the people who work within them. Theories as described in this paper from education and organizational development support the premise that reflection can enable transformative action (Friere 2002; Mezirow 1991; Schön 1991).

Strategic conversations within and across health and social sectors provide individuals with opportunities to co-create a shared vision and co-design a plan forward.

The development of the Ontario IPC Blueprint for Action (IPCSC 2007) provides a concrete example of how system-level conversations can occur to stimulate change. Engagement is a critical factor for success, with strategic opportunities to enable reflection and to support a process of designing future directions. Interprofessional client-centered collaborative care begins with our own willingness to reflect upon our own practices and opportunities for change. These reflective practices must occur at the micro, meso, and macro levels in all healthcare organizations and across the healthcare system to support the cultural shift that has been long desired and is on the road to being achieved!

REFERENCES

Brewer, M. L., & Jones, S. (2013). An interprofessional practice capability framework focusing on safe, high-quality, client-centred health services. *Journal of Allied Health,* 42(2), e45–e49.

Bushe, G.R., & Kassam, A.F. (2005). When is appreciative inquiry transformational? A meta-case analysis. *Journal of Applied Behavioral Science,* 41(2), 161–181. http://dx.doi.org/10.1177/0021886304270337.

Canadian Interprofessional Health Collaborative. (2010). A national interprofessional competency framework. Retrieved from http://www.cihc.ca/files/CIHC_IPCompeten cies_Feb1210.pdf.

Choy, S. (2009).Transformational learning in the workplace.*Journal of Transformative Education,* 7, 64–85. http://dx.doi.org/10.1177/1541 344609334720.

Clark, P. G. (2009). Reflecting on reflection in interprofessional education: Implications for theory and practice. *Journal of Interprofessional Care,* 23, 213–223. http://dx.doi.org/10.1080/13561820902877195.

Coffey, S., & Anyinam, C. (2015). Interprofessional health care practice. Toronto, Canada: Pearson.

College of Family Physicians of Canada. (2011). A vision for Canada: Family practice: The patient's medical home. Retrieved from www.cfpc.ca /uploadedFiles/Resources/ Resource_Items/PMH_A_Vision_for_Canada.pdf.

Cooperrider, D., & Whitney, D. (1999).Collaborating for change: Appreciative inquiry.San Francisco, CA: Barrett-Koehler.

Cranton, P. (2011). A transformative perspective on the scholarship of teaching and learning. Higher Education Research & Development, 30,75–86. http://dx.doi.org/ 10.1080/07294360.2011.536974.

D'Amour, D., & Oandasan, I. (2005). Interprofessionality as the field of interprofessional practice and interprofessional education: An emerging concept. *Journal of Interprofessional Care,* 19(Suppl. 1), 8–20. http://dx.doi.org/10.1080/13561820 500081604.

Davis, K., Schoen, C., & Schoenbaum, S. C. (2000).A 2020 vision for American health care. *Archives of Internal Medicine,* 160, 3357–3362. http://dx.doi.org/10.1001/ archinte.160.22.3357.

D'Eon, M. (2005). A blueprint for interprofessional learning. *Journal of Interprofessional Care,* 19(Suppl. 1), 49–59. http://dx.doi.org/10.1080 /13561820512331350227.

Ezell, M. (2001). Advocacy in the human services. Belmont, CA: Brooks/Cole Thomas Learning.

Friere, P. (2002). Pedagogy of the oppressed. New York, NY: Continuum.

Health Professions Regulatory Advisory Council. (2009). Critical links: Transforming and supporting patient care. Retrieved from http://www.hprac.org/en/reports/resources/ hpraccriticallinksenglishjan_09.pdf.

Herbert, C. (2005). Changing the culture: Interprofessional education for collaborative patient-centred practice in Canada. *Journal of Interprofessional Care,* 19(Suppl. 1), 1–4. http://dx.doi.org/10.1080 /13561820500081539.

Interprofessional Care Advisory Group.(2006).Proceedings report for the summit on advancing interprofessional education and practice, June 14 -15, 2006: Submitted to the Ontario Ministry of Health and Long-Term Care, Healthforce Ontario. Unpublished document.

Interprofessional Care Steering Committee. (2007). Interprofessional care: A blueprint for action in Ontario.Retrieved from https://www. healthforceontario.ca/UserFiles/file/ PolicymakersResearchers/ipc-blueprint-july-2007-en.pdf.

Interprofessional Care Strategic Implementation Committee. (2010). Implementing interprofessional care in Ontario. Retrieved from http://www.healthforceontario.ca/ UserFiles/file/PolicymakersResearchers/ipc-final-report-may-2010-en.pdf.

Interprofessional Education Collaborative Expert Panel. (2011). Core competencies for interprofessional collaborative practice: Report of an expert panel. Retrieved from http://www.aacn.nche.edu/education-resources/ipecreport.pdf.

Institute of Medicine. (2001). Crossing the quality chasm: A new health care system for the 21st century. Washington, DC: Author.

Mann, K., Gordon, J., & MacLeod, A. (2009).Reflection and reflective practice in health professions education: A systematic review. *Advanced in Health Sciences Education,* 14, 595–621. http://dx.doi.org/10.1007 /s10459-007-9090-2.

Marshak, R .J., & Grant, D. (2008). Organization discourse and new organization development practices. *British Journal of Management,* 19, S7–S19. http://dx.doi.org/10.1111/j.1467-8551.2008.00567.x.

Meuser, J., Bean, T., Goldman, J., & Reeves, S. (2006). Family health teams: A new Canadian interprofessional initiative. *Journal of Interprofessional Care,* 20, 436–438. http://dx.doi.org/10.1080/13561820600874726.

Mezirow, J. (1991). Transformative dimensions of adult learning. San Francisco, CA: Jossey-Bass.

Nelson, S., Tassone, M., & Hodges, B.D. (2014).Creating the health care team of the future: The Toronto model for interprofessional education and practice.Ithaca, NY: Cornell University Press.

Oandasan, I. (Producer). (2006). Carole Laurin: Reflections on interprofessional care [DVD]. Available from http://spp.utoronto.ca.

Oandasan, I., & Barker, K. (2003). Educating for advocacy: Exploring the source and substance of community-responsive physicians. *Academic Medicine,* 78(10), S16–S19. http://dx.doi.org/10.1097/00001888-200310001-00006.

Oandasan, I., & Reeves, S. (2005). Key elements of interprofessional education. Part 2: Factors, processes and outcomes. *Journal of Interprofessional Care,* 19(Suppl. 1), 39–48. http://dx.doi.org/10.1080 /13561820500081703.

Oandasan. I., Robinson, J., Bosco, C., Carol, A., Casimiro, L., Dorschner, D., . . . Schwartz, L. (2009). Final report of the IPC Core Competency Working Group to the Interprofessional Care Strategic Implementation Committee. Retrieved from https://www.healthforceontario.ca/UserFiles   /file/PolicymakersResearchers/resource-guide-ipc-competency-nov-2009-en.pdf.

Regulated Health Professions Act, 1991, RSO 1991, c 18 [Ontario]. Retrieved from https://www.canlii.org/en/on/laws/stat/so-1991-c-18/latest/so-1991-c-18.html.

Schein, E. H. (1993). Organizational culture and leadership (2nd ed.). San Francisco, CA: Jossey-Bass.

Schön, D. A. (1991).The reflective practitioner: How professionals think in action. Hants, United Kingdom: Ashgate.

Senge, P.M. (2006). The fifth discipline: The art and practice of the learning organization. New York, NY: Currency-Doubleday.

Tosti, D. T., & Jackson, S. F. (1994, April 5). Organizational alignment: How it works and why it matters. Training Magazine, 8–64.

World Health Organization. (2010). Framework for action on interprofessional education & collaborative practice. Retrieved from http: //whqlibdoc. who.int/hq/2010/WHO_HRH_HPN_10.3_eng.pdf?ua=1.

In: Interprofessional Client-Centred Collaborative Practice   ISBN: 978-1-63483-754-5
Editor: Carole Orchard   © 2015 Nova Science Publishers, Inc.

Chapter 6

ENGAGING HEALTH PROFESSIONALS IN CONTINUING INTERPROFESSIONAL DEVELOPMENT

Jill Thistlethwaite

University of Technology Sydney,
Sydney, Australia

ABSTRACT

Health professionals are required to undergo continuing professional development (CPD) in order to ensure their skills are up to date.

Such CPD is usually uni-professional. In contrast, continuing interprofessional development (CIPD) should involve health professionals who "learn with, from and about each other" (Centre for the Advancement of Interprofessional Education [CAIPE], 2002, para. 2). CIPD is, therefore, shared learning with the aim of improving patient or client care.

There is a lack of robust evidence that CPD (and therefore CIPD) leads to sustained change in practice. However, one review has concluded that there is evidence that interprofessional education (IPE) can create positive interaction while encouraging interprofessional collaboration, and thus improving client care.

There is, as yet, no agreed model of CIPD for optimal learning. To consider how new knowledge through learning may be translated into action, the model of a knowledge cycle is useful.

Prior to CIPD, participants should undergo a needs assessment, bearing in mind that self-assessment is not particularly reliable. For team-based CIPD, the learning outcomes should be defined by the team. There are a number of strategies to help motivate health professionals and teams to engage in CIPD. A useful learning tool is an authentic case for discussion.

Keywords: Lifelong learning, continuing interprofessional development, situated learning, community of practice, participatory learning

INTRODUCTION

In many countries, and for most health professions, practitioners are required to ensure their skills are up to date and to provide evidence of CPD in order to maintain their licensure to practice. In some cases, the evidence may simply be the need to show attendance at relevant courses; in others, proof of learning or change may be required (e.g., through audit or quality improvement processes). Less frequently, certain accreditation bodies in some jurisdictions require a more formal process of recertification or revalidation. However, a commonality is the concept that being, and remaining, a health professional requires lifelong learning and regular up-skilling.

CPD is usually a uni-professional pursuit, or at least there are few requirements for the inclusion of interprofessional development. Each profession has a set number of activities for achieving a requisite number of points, credits, or hours. The activities may be multiprofessional, involving common learning and associated with generic and topic-based learning outcomes. Few CPD offerings involve specific interprofessional learning outcomes and shared learning that is inclusive of "learn[ing] with, from and about each other" (CAIPE 2002, para. 2), which the definition of IPE requires.

The World Health Organization (1998) recommends CIPD to encourage "learning together to work together" (p. 4) amongst health care professionals. The World Health Organization's recommendation that continuing medical education (the term in common usage before CPD) should be broader and involve more than one health profession is not new. Headrick, Wilcock, and Batalden's article in the *British Medical Journal* published in 1998 advocated for a greater emphasis on IPE, suggesting that most health professionals have a motivation to learn in common, and at least one shared value in the desire to provide optimal care to meet the needs of their clients or patients. Therefore, learning together should help health professionals provide answers to "the swampy problems most important to the health of their patients and communities" (Headrick et al. 1998, p. 771).

Evidence for the Effectiveness of CPD

Often CPD is a tick-box exercise with professionals meeting the minimum requirements to adhere to the stated standards. In part, this disillusionment may be due to a perceived lack of evidence regarding the effectiveness of CPD in relation to improving client outcomes. Forsetlund et al.'s (2009) Cochrane review of educational meetings and workshops, which included over 80,000 health professionals in 81 trials, concluded that this type of learning can, in fact, improve client outcomes and positively alter professional practice. However, any learning effect was thought likely to be small and, particularly in relation to changes in complex behaviors, no better than other types of CPD such as audit. A mixture of didactic and interactive activities appeared to be optimal methods, although many of the studies lacked detail about what the interventions consisted of or included (Forsetlund et al. 2009). While Forsetlund et al. focused on continuing medical education, professions other than medicine were included in their review; however, there was no indication that any of the educational input was interprofessional.

Traditionally, CPD for physicians tends to focus on updating knowledge, and thus has not been designed to promote change in behavior. Therefore, educators have suggested that CPD activities should plan input using established theories of behavior change such as sociocultural theories (Légaré et al. 2014). Similar findings have been made in relation to nursing CPD, which has tended to be didactic rather than participatory and realistic (Griscti and Jacono 2006).

Evidence for CIPD as Shared Learning

To fit with the definition of IPE as "learn[ing] with, from and about" (CAIPE 2002, para. 2), any CIPD should be interactive. However, critics of IPE, and those health professionals who prefer to learn with their own in-group, are likely to ask for evidence that such shared interactive learning has any effect on teamwork, patient safety, or organizational change. Reviews examining the effectiveness of IPE have not found any convincing evidence of change in any of these important outcomes overall (Reeves, Perrier, Goldman, Freeth and Zwarenstein 2013).

The World Health Organization's (2010) *Framework for Action on Interprofessional Education and Collaborative Practice* did summarize existing evidence for IPE, but it did not provide a systematic review; this framework has indeed been criticized for not appraising the available evidence (Barr 2010). Reeves et al.'s Cochrane review from 2008 had rigorous inclusion criteria—studies had to report on randomized controlled trials (RCTs), controlled before and after (CBA) studies, and/or interrupted time series (ITS) studies. This resulted in only six studies meeting the criteria: four were RCTs and two CBAs (Reeves et al. 2008). Generalizations are difficult from this review because of the variety of learning outcomes and activities as well as the length of educational interventions and professions involved (Thistlethwaite 2012). However, of interest to CIPD, four papers reviewed in Reeves et al.'s work did provide evidence that IPE in the clinical workplace led to positive outcomes in (a) collaborative team work and subsequent client safety in the emergency department (Morey et al. 2002); (b) care for victims of domestic violence (Thompson et al. 2000); (c) client satisfaction in the emergency department due to change in culture (Campbell et al. 2001); and (d) delivery of care by mental health professionals (Young et al. 2005). An earlier review had wider inclusion criteria and focused less on whether IPE is effective and more on how and why it works and under what circumstances (Barr et al. 2005). Barr et al.'s (2005) review also concluded that there is evidence that IPE creates positive interaction, encourages interprofessional collaboration, and improves client care; however, no agreed model appears to be better than any other.

However, health care providers can also look at the impact of the lack of interprofessional collaboration to satisfy the need for change in CIPD. The importance of interprofessional communication has been highlighted by several failures of client care and safety in the United Kingdom, Australia, and the United States in recent years (e.g., Francis, 2013; Garling 2008).

CIPD to Promote Change

Health care providers know that the transfer of evidence based on research outputs is slow to be incorporated into practice (Morris, Woodings, and Grant 2011). For CIPD to have an effect on practice, health care professionals need to take into account how knowledge is transferred and implemented after any educational intervention (i.e., how knowledge is translated into action). This can happen through the following phases of Graham et al.'s (2006) knowledge cycle:

- Identify the problem—this could be poor interprofessional communication, a dysfunctional team, poor feedback from colleagues or team workers, patient safety adverse events, or lack of client-centered care.
- Identify and review the best available knowledge relevant to the problem—this could be done during the CIPD event or prior by a facilitator and the participants (CIPD preparation).
- Adapt the knowledge selected for the local context—or facilitator preparation.
- Discuss the barriers to applying this knowledge by the participants and identify any organizational factors—this occurs during the CIPD event.
- Discuss and agree on interventions for the local situation to promote the use of the knowledge (and skills) gained—this occurs during the CIPD event.
- Evaluate the outcomes of the intervention in the short and long term (for participants, the organization, and the clients)—organizers of the event carry out short- and long-term evaluation.
- Put measures into place to sustain the change—this involves all participants and their organizations over time.

Identifying the Content for CIPD

Best practice in relation to CPD in general terms should include practitioners considering where their weaknesses lie and their educational needs, perhaps based on significant events in their practice or clients' unmet needs. By reflecting on such a needs assessment, practitioners then decide the optimal way in which to meet those needs. Pragmatically, however, many choose their learning based on courses or activities available at the right time, at a convenient location (which may include online), and for a reasonable price. Moreover, self-evaluation and self-reflection on performance with subsequent self-planning of CPD to enhance performance have been criticized as evidence suggests that self-assessment is rarely accurate (Davis et al. 2006). Therefore, health professionals should not rely solely on their own perceptions of competence or capability (Eva and Regehr 2005). Rather, self-assessment should be integrated with feedback from multiple sources (Eva, Regehr, and Gruppen 2012), and this feedback should enable a dialogue between the provider and the recipient so that the health professional is enabled to work through the feedback and make guided changes (Boud 2015).

A commonly used method of collecting peer and client input is through multisource feedback (MSF). The MSF forms include questions about teamwork, interactions with colleagues from one's own and other professions, communication skills, client-centeredness, and so forth. Specific instruments for client satisfaction, such as patient satisfaction questionnaires, may be utilized and can include questions about client-centered care and how the client and family felt involved in treatment decisions. Although these forms focus on the specific individual rather than a whole team, they may be appropriate if a health professional works across several locations and in different collaborations. For fixed teams, it makes more sense to utilize a team MSF. The team's employer or organization may also be involved in helping decide the focus of the CIPD for that team.

The American Board of Internal Medicine has developed an online tool for physicians to assess their competency in interprofessional teamwork and to compare this with feedback from their colleagues through an MSF process (Chesluk et al. 2015). The teamwork effectiveness assessment module within the American Board of Internal Medicine tool has been piloted by 20 hospital-based medical professionals, who engaged with an average of 13 raters each, most of whom were nurses (Chesluk et al. 2015). The majority of participants were able to identify their team members, assess their own teamwork skills, elicit feedback from their colleagues on these skills, reflect on the feedback, and plan improvements (Chesluk et al. 2015). While such tools are useful, I suggest they be developed for all professions and that there is a danger that very positive feedback is unlikely to motivate physicians to engage in CIPD.

Engaging Busy Professionals

One way to engage professionals in CIPD is to offer team-based education for existing interprofessional teams or collaborations. In team-based CIPD the desired learning outcomes are defined by the team, for the team, following a careful and frank reflection on their teamwork, perhaps with the aid of an external facilitator. However, such CIPD is more likely to be successful if the team is well established and members are used to learning and performing together. Such sessions require dedicated protected time when all the team can learn together, which may be difficult if service delivery continues to be needed. In practice, many professionals work in multiple teams with looser collaborations, and team members may not see the need for interprofessional learning.

To engage professionals in CIPD some or all of the following are likely to be necessary:

- A professional accreditation body or employers must require the professional's CPD include a certain percentage of interprofessional learning.
- Learning outcomes and activities must be relevant to the professional's practice.
- Learning activities must encourage team attendance with the aim of enhancing team performance.
- The session involves significant event analysis or addresses a patient safety problem highlighting poor communications between professional groups.
- The activities include self or external diagnosis of dysfunctional team behavior.
- Professionals have experience with interprofessional conflict and be willing to change to avoid or prevent such conflict in the future.

- The organization must offer protected time for team learning so that all team members may be present.
- It is beneficial if professionals have prior experience of useful and engaging IPE.

It is vitally important for CIPD to define clearly what the learning outcomes for participants are and to include those that may only be achieved through interprofessional interaction (see Box 1). If the learning outcomes are not appropriate or relevant to every professional, potential participants may question the need to learn together.

Rather than didactic processes to aid knowledge acquisition, current thinking is that professional development should be based on adult learning principles (see Box 2). Empirical research has shown that effective learning is optimally undertaken within a community supportive of professional learning; such situated learning helps professionals engage with the process of actively working with others on authentic problems (Webster-Wright 2009). Situated learning is the process of learning from one's environment, interactions, and work and social contexts. Thus, CPD should ideally be continuing, social, interactive, and professionally relevant (Webster-Wright 2009). A commonly used term for this process of learning that may be applied to interprofessional and collaborative learning activities is "community of practice" (Lave and Wenger 1991, p. 29).

Box 1. Examples of learning outcomes for a team-based learning activity

- An understanding of an agreement on the team's values.
- An understanding of an agreement on the nature and practice of being client centered.
- Exploration and discussion of team members' roles and responsibilities.
- Recommendations for any necessary changes in how the team works together.
- Negotiation and conflict resolution skills.

Box 2. Principles of adult learning

- As adults are autonomous and self-directed, they should be encouraged to set their own learning outcomes; however, for CIPD, the learning outcomes are best set as a group process.
- Didactic input should be kept to a minimum—only frame the parameters of interactive discussion.
- Learning is best built on participants' experiences and their existing knowledge; they should connect the learning activity to their current situation and skills.
- Adults are goal orientated; they need to know the defined learning outcomes and the purpose of the CIPD.
- Adult learners require time for feedback and reflective dialogue.
- All professionals should be treated as equals, show and be shown respect.

Such participatory learning involves small group activities and time for reflection on group or team processes during learning. The theories of teamwork, team function, client centeredness, and collaborative practice need to be aligned with the practical—what happens, or what should happen, in health care delivery. As health professionals learn together, they each bring a fount of experience and narratives; these shared experiences should inform the learning, building on what participants already know but may wish to improve or change. When working through an activity, learning is more powerful if the activity is based on examples from group participants. When the participants are from an actual health care team, they can be facilitated to work through examples of current or past experiences. These experiences may be near misses or significant events, but also should include times when the team worked well together to reflect on why and how this happens (see Box 3).

Box 3. Trigger questions for discussions about significant events

- What happened?
- What have you/the team learnt from this incident?
- How might things have been done differently?
- How might the team improve following this incident and the discussion?
- What is the benefit of discussing incidents like this?

Use of a Case Study to Stimulate Discussion: The Case of Martha Schmidt

 Martha Schmidt is a 60-year-old woman who completed her university degree in library science and has worked as a librarian part time in the local library for the past 35 years, only taking time off when she had each of her three children (now 28, 30, and 32 years of age). She is married to Thomas who is 61 years old.

Martha has suffered from anxiety bouts over the past decade, which caused high blood pressure, and recently she suffered a cerebral vascular accident (i.e., a stroke), which resulted in mild cognitive deficits and some right-sided arm and leg weakness. She returned home shortly after having the stroke, but this change in her abilities has had a profound effect on her. She is right-side dominant and has also experienced some visual changes that have incapacitated her and caused her to worry about whether she will be able to return to her part-time work that she loves.

Martha has always been involved in her community's activities, including being part of a book club, the quilting group, and a key member of the group that helps to set up an annual summer fair baking contest. Martha loves cooking and baking, and this love has resulted in her putting on weight over the past several years to the point now where she is carrying 175 pounds on her 5-foot-5-inch frame. She has frequently said that she wants to become more active, but has not found the motivation to change from her current low activity level. Her family physician had also cautioned her about her blood pressure and high cholesterol levels but with little impact.

Her stroke was a real wake-up call for her, and unfortunately there was a delay in initiating treatment that has left her with impairments. Martha worries about how Thomas will be able to accept these changes in her abilities. He loves to golf in the spring, summer, and fall and to ski in the winter. Hence he is quite active. Thomas also has a university degree in business management and is currently the town's bank manager at the Royal Bank branch.

Thomas has seen big changes in Martha since her stroke and worries about how she can manage for herself when he is at work and out golfing or skiing. He has noted she sometimes has trouble following his conversations with her, which is very stressful, as he loved the deep discussions they used to have about books they were both reading. He worries as well if their home is suitable for Martha, as he has noticed how hard it is for her to manage the stairs to the 2nd floor. They have always had a cleaning lady so this has helped with Martha's adjustment to her new situation.

However, things she used to do independently like bathing and grooming herself, making meals, and driving to the local grocery store now require assistance.

Martha can no longer drive her car and must rely on her two daughters or Thomas to take her now. These changes are real challenges for her. Martha has always loved being a mother. She has a loving, warm relationship with her adult daughters who live within a 1- to 2-hour drive of her home. Her 28-year-old daughter, Sharon, has always been dependent on her mother's advice and direction. Sharon completed a dental assistant diploma at the nearby community college, and she currently works full time in a dental office as a dental assistant and, like her mother, has a weight problem. Sharon is tall (5'10") and 250 lbs. Martha and Thomas' son, Daniel, is 30 years of age and is employed in Afghanistan with the Canadian Armed Forces. He occasionally calls home to connect with the family. Martha's other daughter, Karen, who is 32 years of age, obtained a police foundations diploma from the same community college as Sharon and currently works full time as an Ontario Provincial Policewoman. She, like Sharon, is very close to her mother, and all three women often went out together on outings. Sharon and Karen have had trouble coming to terms with the changes in their mother following her stroke.

Karen has recently become engaged to another Ontario Provincial Police officer, and she was looking forward to planning her forthcoming wedding with her mother. The stroke changes all her plans. She has had to delay the wedding while coming to terms with her mother's change in physical and cognitive capacities.

Although the family members are all experiencing stress and deep sadness over the changes in Martha, they have been reluctant to sit down together and discuss how they are feeling.

Note. From *Grey Bruce Case Study – The Case of Martha Schmidt* (p. 1), by the Stroke Network Southwestern Ontario and University of Western Ontario, 2015. Retrieved from http://www.ipe.uwo.ca/Administration/Grey%20Bruce%20Case%20Study.pdf

A case such as that of Martha is an ideal trigger for discussion of interprofessional client-centered collaborative practice. The case should be written with the team and health professionals attending the CIPD in mind, or the team itself may present a client narrative that that they wish to discuss in more detail.

With a written case, it would also be effective to have a simulated client play the role. This enables the portrayal of a more authentic scenario in which the simulated client and simulated carers (as well as family members as appropriate) bring to life ideas, concerns, expectations, and values.

For Martha's case, the participants can discuss Martha's needs and priorities and the best approach to meet these. They should decide on a management plan and timeline, taking into account team members' roles and capabilities.

An Example of a Team Management Plan for Martha and Her Family

For each individual client case, the team of health professionals has to welcome the client (and other relevant individuals) into the team—this is the meaning of the 'client at the center of the team.' The plan, therefore, is discussed and agreed upon in collaboration with Martha and her family members.

Martha's priorities, her family's priorities, and the health professionals' priorities may not be aligned.

The plan should include a consideration of Martha's medical, psychological, social and, if appropriate, spiritual needs.

Health professionals should also be considerate of the family's finances and aware of the support available in a particular location; for example, subsidized health and social services will differ across national as well as provincial and state boundaries.

The following areas are likely to be priorities (and all interact holistically):

- Physical assessment, including mobility and activities of daily living, diet, and physical activity;
- Cognitive assessment (i.e., determine why Martha appears to have difficulties in conversation);
- Psychological assessment (i.e., evaluate how Martha is adjusting to her changed health status);
- Home environment (i.e., determine how this may be improved);
- Community assessment (i.e., explore available services and assess the level of social support Martha has from her friends); and
- Medication review.

Each of the above priorities may involve different health professionals, so there is also a need for interprofessional communication and to ensure that care does not become fragmented.

Ideally, a nominated professional oversees Martha's management plan and is the first point of contact for Martha and her family.

CONCLUSION

The following list presents a summary of key points relating to CIPD:

- CIPD should involve specific interprofessional learning outcomes and shared learning, inclusive of "learn[ing] with, from and about each other" (CAIPE, 2002, para. 2).
- CIPD activities should be planned using established theories of behavior change such as sociocultural theories.
- At this point, no agreed model appears to be better than any other for CIPD.
- By use of a needs assessment, practitioners decide what their learning needs are and how they may be met.
- Self-evaluation and self-reflection on performance with subsequent self-planning of CIPD to enhance performance are rarely accurate; therefore, self-assessment should be integrated with feedback from multiple sources (i.e., MSF).
- In team-based CIPD, the desired learning outcomes are defined by the team for the team, following a careful and frank reflection on their teamwork, perhaps with the aid of an external facilitator.
- Learning outcomes and activities should be relevant to professionals' practices.
- If the learning outcomes are not appropriate or relevant to every professional, potential participants may question the need to learn together.

CIPD should be planned with adult learning principles in mind. Ideally, such participatory learning involves small group activities and time for reflection on group or team processes during learning.

REFERENCES

Barr, H. (2010). Commentary: The WHO framework for action. *Journal of Interprofessional Care, 24*, 475–478. http://dx.doi.org/10.3109/13561820.2010.504134.

Barr, H., Koppel, I., Reeves, S., Hammick, M., and Freeth, D. (2005). *Effective interprofessional education: Assumption, argument and evidence.* London, United Kingdom: Blackwell.

Boud, D. (2015). Feedback: Ensuring that it leads to enhanced learning. *The Clinical Teacher, 12*, 3–7. http://dx.doi.org/10.1111/tct.12345.

Campbell, J. C., Coben, J. H., McLoughlin, E., Dearwater, S., Nah, G., Glass, N., . . . Durborow, N. (2001). An evaluation of a system-change training model to improve emergency department response to battered women. *Academic Emergency Medicine, 8*, 131–138. http://dx.doi.org/10.1111/j.1553-2712.2001.tb01277.x.

Centre for the Advancement of Interprofessional Education. (2002). *Defining IPE.* Retrieved from http://www.CAIPE.org.uk/about-us/defining-ipe/

Chesluk, B. J., Reddy, S., Hess, B., Bernabeo, E., Lynn, L., and Holmboe, E. (2015). Assessing interprofessional teamwork: Pilot test of a new assessment model for practicing physicians. *Journal of Continuing Education in the Health Professions, 35*, 3–10. http://dx.doi.org/10.1002/chp.21267.

Davis, D. A., Mazmanian, P., Fordis, M., Van Harrison, R., Thorpe, K. E., and Perrier, L. (2006). Accuracy of physician self-assessment compared with observed measures of competence. *JAMA, 296*, 1094–1102. http://dx.doi.org/10.1001/jama.296.9.1094.

Eva, K. W., and Regehr, G. (2005). Self-assessment in the health professions: A reformulation and research agenda. *Academic Medicine, 80*, S46–S54.

Eva, K. W., Regehr, G., and Gruppen, L. (2012). Blinded by "insight": Self-assessment and its role in performance improvement. In B. D. Hodges and L. Lingard (Eds.), *The question of competence* (pp. 131–154). Ithaca, NY: ILR Press.

Forsetlund, L., Bjørndal, A., Rashidian, A., Jamtvedt, G., O'Brien, M. A., Wolf, F. M., . . . Oxman, A. D. (2009). Continuing education meetings and workshops: Effects on professional practice and health care outcomes (Review). *Cochrane Database of Systematic Reviews, 2*, Art. No. CD003030. http://dx.doi.org/10.1002/14651858.CD003030.pub2.

Francis, R. (2013). *Report of the Mid Staffordshire NHS Foundation Trust public inquiry.* London, United Kingdom: The Stationary Office.

Garling, P. (2008). *Final report of the special commission of inquiry: Acute care services in NSW public hospitals.* New South Wales, Australia: State of NSW through the Special Commission of Inquiry.

Graham, I. D, Logan, J., Harrison, M. B., Straus, S. E., Tetroe, J., Caswell, W., and Robinson, N. (2006). Lost in knowledge translation: Time for a map? *Journal of Continuing Education in the Health Professions, 26*, 13–24. http://dx.doi.org/10.1002/chp.47.

Griscti, O., and Jacono, J. (2006). Effectiveness of continuing education programmes in nursing: Literature review. *Journal of Advanced Nursing, 55,* 449–456. http://dx.doi.org/10.1111/j.1365-2648.2006.03940.x.

Headrick, L. A., Wilcock, P. M., and Batalden, P. B (1998). Interprofessional working and continuing medical education. *BMJ, 316,* 771. http://dx.doi.org/10.1136/bmj.316.7133.771.

Lave, J., and Wenger, E. (1991). *Situated learning: Legitimate peripheral participation.* Cambridge, United Kingdom: Cambridge University Press.

Légaré, F., Freitas, A., Thompson-Leduc, P., Borduas, F., Luconi, F., Boucher, A., Jacques, A. (2014). The majority of accredited continuing professional development activities do not target clinical behaviour change. *Academic Medicine, 90,* 197–202. http://dx.doi.org/10.1097/ACM.0000000000000543.

Morey, J. C., Simon, R., Jay, G. D., Wears, R. L., Salisbury, M., Dukes, K. A., and Burns, S. D. (2002). Error reduction and performance improvement in the emergency department through formal teamwork training: Evaluation results of the MedTeams project. *Health Services Research, 37,* 1553–1581. http://dx.doi.org/10.1111/1475-6773.01104.

Morris, Z. S., Woodings, S., and Grant, J. (2011). The answer is 17 years, what is the question: Understanding time lags in translational research. *Journal of the Royal Society of Medicine, 104,* 510–520. http://dx.doi.org/10.1258/jrsm.2011.110180.

Reeves, S., Perrier, L. Goldman, J., Freeth, D., and Zwarenstein, M. (2013).). Interprofessional education: Effects on professional practice and health care outcomes (update) (review). The Cochrane Collaboration. Issue 3. http//www.thecochranelibrary.com.

Reeves, S., Zwarenstein, M., Goldman, J., Barr, H., Freeth, D., Hammick, M., and Koppel, I. (2008). Interprofessional education: Effects on professional practice and health care outcomes. *Cochrane Database of Systematic Reviews* 2008, *1,* Art. No. CD002213. http://dx.doi.org/10.1002/14651858.CD002213.pub2.

Thistlethwaite, J. E. (2012). Interprofessional education: A review of context, learning and the research agenda. *Medical Education, 46,* 58–70. http://dx.doi.org/10.1111/j.1365-2923.2011.04143.x.

Thompson, R. S., Rivara, F. P., Thompson, D. C., Barlow, W. E., Sugg, N. K., Maiuro, R. D., and Rubanowice, D. M. (2000). Identification and management of domestic violence: A randomized trial. *American Journal of Preventative Medicine, 19,* 253–263. http://dx.doi.org/10.1016/S0749-3797(00)00231-2.

Webster-Wright, A. (2009). Reframing professional development through understanding authentic professional development. *Review of Educational Research, 79,* 702–739. http://dx.doi.org/10.3102/0034654308330970.

World Health Organization. (1988). *Learning together to work together for health* (Technical Report Series 769). Retrieved from http://whqlibdoc.who.int/trs/WHO_TRS_769.pdf.

World Health Organization. (2010). *Framework for action on interprofessional education and collaborative practice.* Retrieved from http://whqlibdoc.who.int/hq/2010/WHO_HRH_HPN_10.3_eng.pdf?ua=1

Young, A. S., Chinman, M., Forquer, S. L., Knight, E. L., Vogel, H., Miller, A., . . . Mintz, J. (2005). Use of a consumer-led intervention to improve provider competencies. *Psychiatric Services, 56,* 967–975. http://dx.doi.org/10.1176/appi.ps.56.8.967.

In: Interprofessional Client-Centred Collaborative Practice   ISBN: 978-1-63483-754-5
Editor: Carole Orchard   © 2015 Nova Science Publishers, Inc.

Chapter 7

THE EFFECT OF LEADERSHIP SUPPORT ON INTERPROFESSIONAL PRACTICE, TEAM EFFECTIVENESS, AND PATIENT SAFETY OUTCOMES

Heather K. S. Laschinger[1], Brenda J. Stutsky[2] and Emily A. Read[1]

[1]Arthur Labatt Family School of Nursing, Western University,
London, ON, Canada
[2]University of Manitoba, Faculty of Medicine,
Division of Continuing Professional Development,
Winnipeg, MN, Canada

ABSTRACT

Patient safety is an essential component of high quality health care that is influenced by interprofessional collaboration (IPC). Leaders are thought to play a critical role in shaping health care work environments that support IPC and patient safety, yet few empirical studies have tested these relationships. The purpose of this study was to test a theoretical model linking leadership support for IPC to health professionals' perceptions of interprofessional collaboration, team effectiveness, and perceptions of patient safety in health care settings. A cross-sectional survey of 116 health care providers from Manitoba, Canada, was conducted. Descriptive statistics were analyzed using SPSS. Structural equation modeling with maximum likelihood estimation in Amos was used to test the hypothesized model. The model fit was acceptable: $\chi^2(129) = 193.02$; $\chi^2/df = 1.50$; CFI = .92; IFI = .92; RMSEA = .066 and the relationships between variables were significant and in the expected direction. Findings showed that leaders who support IPC by providing access to formalized support structures that facilitate collaboration and communication among team members have a positive effect on IPC, which in turn have positive effects on team effectiveness and patient safety. Leadership support for IPC is an important factor that influences team effectiveness and patient safety. Creating the necessary workplace conditions for health care providers to engage in IPC is one way that leaders can positively influence patient safety within health care organizations.

Keywords: Leadership, interprofessional collaboration, patient safety, team effectiveness

INTRODUCTION

Patient safety is a fundamental component of high quality health care delivery to patients (World Health Organization 2006). The Institute of Medicine (IOM) identified patient safety as a key priority for health care systems, resulting in systematic efforts to reduce the risks to which patients are exposed in health care settings (Kohn, Corrigan, and Donaldson 1999; Page 2003). The IOM landmark report *To Err is Human* (Kohn et al. 1999) estimated that up to 98,000 patients in the United States die each year because of adverse events. Similar results were found in a Canadian study (Baker et al. 2004, p. 1683). Annual costs of adverse events are estimated to cost approximately $1.1 billion in Canada (Etchells et al. 2012) and the US (David, Gunnarsson, Waters, Horblyuk, and Kaplan 2013). Research is needed to understand factors responsible for the human and system costs of unsafe patient care.

Effective collaboration within interprofessional teams seems to be associated with improvements in patient safety (Kohn et al. 1999). Collaborative practice is defined by the World Health Organization (2010) as occurring "when multiple health workers from different professional backgrounds provide comprehensive services by working with patients, their families, carers and communities to deliver the highest quality of care across settings" (p. 13). Teamwork among health care team members plays an important causal role in preventing adverse patient outcomes (Mansour 2009), highlighting the importance of IPC for patient safety.

Transformational leadership which has been shown to support shared leadership in teamwork has been identified as an important mechanism for developing supportive work environments that, in turn, promote patient safety (p. 2003). The purpose of the study described in this chapter was to test a theoretical model linking leadership support for IPC to health professionals' perceptions of interprofessional collaboration, team effectiveness, and patient safety in health care settings.

Theoretical Framework

According to Stutsky and Laschinger (2014), interprofessional collaborative practice (IPC) is influenced by situational factors in health care work settings, such as leadership efforts to foster IPC and formalized IPC support structures embedded in the system. IPC, in turn, results in greater team effectiveness and higher perceptions of patient safety (see Figure VII). In Stutsky's framework, interprofessional collaboration is characterized by four dimensions: *collective ownership of goals, understanding of team member roles, interdependent working relationships,* and *ongoing knowledge exchange* (Stutsky and Laschinger 2014). Collective ownership of goals refers to a shared responsibility among team members for setting and working towards team objectives (D'Amour, Goulet, Labadie, San Martín-Rodriguez, and Pineault 2008). Understanding roles refers to health care providers' knowledge and understanding of team member roles and responsibilities (Canadian Interprofessional Health Collaborative 2010). Interdependence refers to the degree to which team members' work is connected with that of others, through cooperation and communication among members to accomplish work goals (Canadian Health Services Research Foundation 2006). Finally, knowledge exchange refers to the extent to which information sharing between health providers occurs in the workplace (D'Amour et al. 2008; Safran, Miller, and Beckman 2006).

IPC is influenced by leader support for development of and communication of clear goals and expectations among health care team members in the practice setting that create conditions for effective collaboration (Temkin-Greener, Gross, Kunitz, and Mukamel 2004).

Formalized workplace support structures, such as, physical space, time, policies and procedures, provide a supportive infrastructure intended to optimize IPC. Leaders play a key role in ensuring these IPC support structures are in place.

Strong leadership is needed to manage the complexity of interprofessional teamwork by bringing team members together in constructive and complimentary ways that enhance overall team effectiveness and promote high quality patient care. Shortell, Rousseau, Gillies, Devers, and Simons (1991) found that team leader behaviors influenced health care team dynamics by setting social norms and expectations through their own actions. Both leadership and team functioning have been identified as key competencies of IPC (Bainbridge, Nasmith, Orchard, and Wood 2010). Therefore further understanding of how leadership practices can positively influence IPC in health care teams is important.

Researchers examining the effects of formal leaders on interprofessional health care teams found that relational-focused leadership styles such as authentic leadership are associated with higher levels of interprofessional collaboration (Laschinger and Smith 2013; Regan, Laschinger, and Wong 2015) and unit-level effectiveness (Laschinger, Read, Wilk, and Finegan 2014). Leaders also exert their influence on team effectiveness through support of group processes such as communication, coordination, and conflict management. For example, Temkin-Greener et al. (2004) found that leadership was significantly associated with team cohesion, which in turn influenced team effectiveness.

Leaders can also influence IPC by developing specific skills that make them more effective when leading interprofessional health care teams. For example, in a qualitative study of health care leaders, Stiles, Horton-Deutsch, and Andrews (2014) found that more successful interprofessional leaders were those who intentionally developed new skills that allowed them to be effective in their roles, such as understanding group dynamics, appreciating team member contributions, engaging in self-reflection, and being willing to consider multiple points of view. Curran (2006) maintains that senior management funding for teamwork skill development is critical to foster a culture of IPC in health care organizations. Hence, to be successful IPC must be overtly valued at all levels of organizational leadership. Overt leadership valuing requires "words and deeds by a leader or leaders that indicate an invitation and appreciation for others' contributions" (Nembhard and Edmonson 2006, p. 947). When present, health care professionals experienced feelings of positive psychological safety and subsequent engagement in quality improvement activities. This suggests that one mechanism through which leaders foster IPC is by creating a psychologically safe workplace for all members of an interprofessional health care team.

Leaders accomplish this by being democratic and supportive, welcoming questions and challenges from those they lead, and recognizing the efforts of all team members in accomplishing team goals. Overall, these findings show that developing positive relationships with those they lead is a central role of leaders of interprofessional health care teams.

Leaders face challenges in their efforts to promote IPC among team members including varying professional roles and responsibilities, priorities, and professional cultures (Hall 2005; Reeves, MacMillan, and van Soeren 2010). These diverse perspectives often lead to conflicts within teams. Mitchell, Parker, Giles, and Boyle (2014) found that the degree of conflict associated with diverse teams was stronger for team members with greater professional identification leading to reduced openness to others' perspectives and ideas. Differences between team members' power and status may also contribute to relational difficulties in interprofessional teams. Most notably, studies have shown the traditional medical model supporting care decision making by physicians only still tends to dominate patient care priorities (Reeves et al. 2010).

The implementation of IPC necessitates that team members work together and equally value each other's input with the resulting outcome being shared decision making. However, the formally approved patient decision making models in health agencies prevent this shared approach. This lack of openness for relevant health professionals to be able to make care decisions has the potential to limit acceptance of IPC. Lingard et al. (2012) found that while most health care professionals valued IPC and shared leadership, physicians tended to engage in behaviors that supported the traditional physician-dominated hierarchy in health care. Interestingly in other studies, while physicians thought that they were collaborative and egalitarian, other team members did not always share this perception. Nembhard and Edmonson (2006) found a status gradient in psychological safety among team members, which may account for physician dominance on health care teams. Leaders see the need for a systematic approach to changing current approaches to care to a more participative, interdependent collaborative approach that is rewarded within the system (Curran, 2005).

Overall, these findings suggest that actualizing IPC may be difficult to enact if health care professionals choose to prioritize their own professional perspectives without considering the viewpoints of others. Thus there is an urgent need for leaders desiring to facilitate IPC to focus on bringing people together, encouraging openness and sharing of perspectives, and focusing on shared objectives to create positive relationships among interprofessional team members.

Thus, the way that leaders structure the workplace in a manner conducive to collaboration among health care providers will influence IPC. Protected time for interprofessional patient rounds and meetings, meeting space for such activities, and opportunities to set and evaluate shared team goals are some of the ways that leaders can create workplace conditions that support IPC (San Martín-Rodríguez, Beaulieu, D'Amour, and Ferrada Videla 2005). Such structures align with Kanter's (1977, 1993) concept of structural empowerment, that is, employees need access to information, resources, support, and opportunities to learn and grow in order to accomplish their work effectively. In other words, IPC support structures can be viewed as empowering conditions for IPC. Past research has shown that the more general notion of structural empowerment (Laschinger and Smith 2013; Regan et al. 2015) and IPC support structures (Stutsky and Laschinger 2014) are significant predictors of nurses' perceptions of interprofessional collaboration. It can be extrapolated that the same effects are likely to be found among other health professionals working within the same work environment as nurses. These findings may support the theoretical relationship between how workplaces are structured and the degree of IPC within health care teams.

Access to support structures for IPC is therefore an important, but perhaps overlooked, way in which leaders can encourage and support IPC among their health professional teams.

By providing access to support structures for IPC, health professionals will have a greater chance of coordinating their schedules to meet up to discuss patient care needs, plans, and progress. Since there is a high level of interdependence among many health care professionals' roles, this could result in more timely treatments, referrals, or appointments, as well as reduced duplication of services. Service duplications sometimes happen when multiple care providers are trying to help the same patient. Having access to meeting space represents a crucial support structure that provides health care providers with private, protected space to meet and communicate with one another. This allows them to move out of busy public hallways, patient rooms (usually shared), and staff break rooms, which are not conducive to confidentiality or focused discussions. Institutional provision of IPC support structures allow leaders to demonstrate their commitment to IPC and help establish positive group norms towards collaboration.

Based on this reasoning, we hypothesized that leaders influence IPC by providing support structures (H1). In addition, we reasoned that support structures serve as a mechanism through which leadership influences IPC in the workplace. Thus we hypothesized that IPC support structures mediate the relationship between supportive leadership and IPC (H2).

IPC is posited to result in greater teamwork and logically, safer patient care. The link between a health care team's ability to work together (i.e., team processes) and their performance is well-established across a variety of clinical and practice settings. For example, in a study by Poulton and West (1999) of primary care teams found that team processes such as having shared objectives and team participation were significantly related to team effectiveness and patient-centered care. Interdisciplinary forums for discussion of patient cases have been shown to enhance teamwork and patient-centered care among interprofessional health care teams (Lown and Manning 2010). Studies of surgical teams have shown that teams who engage in frequent information sharing during surgery are less likely to make life-threatening errors (Mazzocco et al. 2009). These studies show that the ability of health care team members to communicate effectively with one another influences the effectiveness of that team and the quality of patient care that they are able to deliver and reduces errors.

Several studies have shown that interventions to develop IPC skills and competence have positive effects on interprofessional teams and better patient outcomes (Salas et al. 2008; Zwarenstein, Goldman, and Reeves 2009). These include practice-based interventions such as daily interprofessional rounds, which have been linked to shorter lengths of stay and lower costs. Deneckere et al. (2013) found that other IPC strategies such as the implementation of care pathways developed within teams resulted in better conflict management, improved organization of patient care, higher competence, and lower burnout levels among interprofessional health care teams working in acute care hospitals. These studies provide encouraging support for the notion that interventions targeting positive attitudes towards IPC competencies can be effective. Based on these findings we hypothesized that higher levels of IPC would be positively related to higher perceptions of team effectiveness (H3).

Patient safety is an important goal of IPC. It makes sense that when health care team members collaborate effectively, patient care quality and patient safety will be addressed and health care providers will be less distracted by team conflicts or misunderstandings (Goh, Chan, and Kuziemsky 2013). Alarmingly, high levels of interprofessional conflict have been associated with increased numbers of significant medical errors (Baldwin and Daugherty 2008), highlighting the potential consequences of poor IPC on patient safety.

Teamwork and collaboration have been identified as key components of a patient safety culture which describes health care organizations that prioritize collective objectives that enhance patient safety including nonpunitive reporting of medication errors and identifying proactive ways to address potential hazards (Goh et al. 2013). Health care leaders play an important role in creating positive patient safety cultures that support IPC. Cheater, Hearnshaw, Baker, and Keane (2005) found that interprofessional meetings resulted in more frequent use of patient safety practices, such as, audit activity and quality improvement efforts to patient care. Raab, Will, Richards, and O'Mara (2013) also found significant improvements in both collaboration and patient safety activities after implementing a comprehensive interprofessional education initiative. Therefore more research testing on relationships between IPC, team effectiveness, and patient safety is needed.

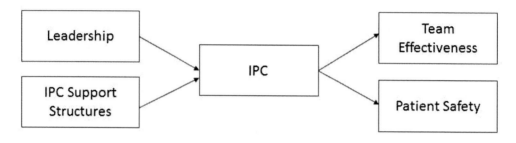

Figure VII. Overall study model.

METHODS

A cross-sectional survey design was used to test the hypothesized model. The sample included 116 health care professionals employed in a regional health authority in northern Manitoba, Canada. Sites included three hospitals, three long-term care facilities, and four primary health care centers. Participants were regulated health care providers who were direct care providers or directly supervised direct care providers.

Procedure

Following ethical approval, questionnaire packages were distributed through the internal mailing systems participating organizations. Completion of the survey constituted consent to participate. An incentive for survey completion included a $2.00 gift card. The anonymous surveys were returned directly to the research team.

The response rate was 32%. Respondents were mostly female (95), ranging from 23 to 68 years of age ($M = 43.40$, $SD = 11.77$), with 0.5 to 40 years of nursing experience ($M = 15.51$, $SD = 12.45$). Seventy-five percent were nurses (i.e., registered nurses, licensed practical nurses, registered psychiatric nurses), 17.2% were allied health professionals (e.g., pharmacists, occupational therapists, physical therapists, social workers, dieticians, and mental health clinicians), and 6.9% were physicians. The majority worked in acute care (57.8%), with 33.6% working in community care, and 6.9% in long-term care.

The majority (71.6%) worked full-time, the remainder worked either part-time (24.1%) or casual (4.3%). The majority (76.7%) had direct patient care roles, 12.9% provided direct care support, and 9.5% were in clinical leadership roles (see Figure VIII).

Demographic Characteristic	N	%	
Profession			
Nurses	87	75.0	
Physician	8	6.9	
Allied Health Professional	20	17.2	
Gender			
Male	21	81.9	
Female	95	18.1	
Highest Level of Education			
Professional Diploma	44	37.9	
Bachelor's Degree	52	44.8	
Master's Degree	7	6.0	
Medical Degree	8	6.9	
Certificate	5	4.3	
Primary Work Setting			
Acute Care	67	57.8	
Community Care	39	33.6	
Long-Term Care	8	6.9	
Primary Work Role			
Direct Patient Care	89	76.7	
Direct Care Support	15	12.9	
Leadership for Direct Care Providers	11	9.5	
Current employment status			
Full Time	83	71.6	
Part Time	28	24.1	
Casual	5	4.3	
	N	Mean	SD
Age	103	43.40	11.77
Years of experience in current role	114	15.51	12.45

Figure VIII. Participant Characteristics.

Instruments

Leadership. Perceptions of leadership were measured using five items based on Temkin-Greener et al.'s (2004) work. Nurses were asked to rate their team leader's ability to facilitate interprofessional collaboration on the unit (e.g., "The team leader fosters professionals from different disciplines to work together"). Items were rated on a 5-point Likert scale from 1 = strongly disagree to 5 = strongly agree). In the current study Cronbach's α was .77.

Support structures. Subscales for support structures, the job characteristics that enable interprofessional collaboration to happen, were based on Parker Oliver, Wittenberg-Lyles, and Day's (2007) work and The Ottawa Hospital Inter-Professional Model of Patient Care Staff Survey (Ottawa Hospital 2007). This scale consisted of five items rated on a 5-point Likert scale from 1 = strongly disagree to 5 = strongly agree, with 1 item being reverse-scored. The instrument had a Cronbach's α of .76 in the current study.

Interprofessional collaboration. The Interprofessional Collaborative Practice Survey developed by Stutsky and Laschinger (2014) was used to measure team members' perceptions of four components of interprofessional collaboration: interdependence (3 items), understanding of roles (3 items), collective ownership of goals (4 items), and ongoing knowledge exchange (4 items). This self-report questionnaire was derived from existing standardized measures that were adapted to be relevant to the health care context. Items for collective ownership of goals, understanding of roles, and interdependence were based on Parker Oliver et al.'s (2007) Modified Index for Interdisciplinary Collaboration while Gaboury, Lapierre, Boon, and Moher's (2011) research provided the basis for the knowledge exchange items.

All items were rated on a 5-point Likert scale from 1 = strongly disagree to 5 = strongly agree. A total score for IPC was calculated by summing and averaging the 14 items in the scale. Higher scores indicate higher levels of interprofessional collaboration. In the current study the Cronbach's α for this total IPC score was .79, demonstrating support for the internal consistency of this measure.

Team effectiveness. Perceived team effectiveness was measured using three items from Temkin-Greener et al.'s (2004) measure of health care professionals' perceptions of their team's ability to meet patient and family needs. Items were rated on a 5-point Likert scale from 1 = strongly disagree to 5 = strongly agree. In the current study the Cronbach's α was .84.

Patient safety. Perceptions of patient safety were assessed using a single item, "Overall, how would you rate the state of patient safety in your clinical area?" from The Ottawa Hospital Inter-Professional Model of Patient Care Staff Survey (Ottawa Hospital 2007). This item has been significantly associated with leadership, empowerment, interprofessional collaborative practice, and team effectiveness (Stutsky and Laschinger 2014).

Data Analysis

Descriptive statistics were done using the Statistical Package for the Social Sciences (SPSS) statistical program (version 22.0, IBM 2014a). Structural equation modeling with maximum likelihood estimation in Amos software (version 22.0, IBM 2014b) was used to examine proposed relationships in the model.

RESULTS

Descriptive Results

Descriptive statistics of major study variables are shown in Figure ix. Perceptions of leadership were moderate, averaging 3.43 on a 5-point scale. Support structures were also moderate (3.25 out of 5). The overall IPC score was 3.75. Of the four IPC components, participants rated interdependence most highly (4.23 out of 5), followed by knowledge exchange (3.86), collective goals (3.49), and understanding roles (3.42). Perceived team effectiveness and patient safety were also rated moderately (3.71 and 3.80 on a 5-point scale, respectively).

Intercorrelations among the model variables are presented in Figure ix. The total IPC scale was significantly correlated with other model variables (r = .42 to .74). The four components of IPC were significantly correlated with one another (r = .27 to .38), and to team effectiveness (r = .25 to .64) and patient safety (r = 29 to .51).

Leadership had moderately positive associations with understanding roles (.29), collective goals (.40), and knowledge exchange (.35), but not with interdependence (r = .11). Support structures were significantly related to all four aspects of IPC (collective ownership of goals, understanding of team member roles, interdependent working relationships, and ongoing knowledge exchange) (range, r = .28 to .44). Finally, perceived team effectiveness was significantly related to patient safety (.55).

Variable	Mean	SD	α	1	2	3	4	5	6	7	8
1. Leadership	3.43	.68	.77	-							
2. Support Structures	3.25	.81	.76	.42	-						
3. Total IPC	3.75	.43	.79	.42	.56	-					
4. Interdependence	4.23	.47	.54	.11	.28	.65	-				
5. Understanding Roles	3.42	.76	.65	.29	.43	.74	.30	-			
6. Collective Goals	3.49	.68	.76	.40	.44	.74	.32	.33	-		
7. Knowledge Exchange	3.86	.48	.55	.35	.41	.66	.38	.27	.36	-	
8. Perceived Team Effectiveness	3.71	.72	.84	.43	.49	.64	.25	.45	.54	.64	-
9. Perceived Patient Safety	3.80	.89	N/A	.24	.36	.51	.29	.35	.40	.51	.55

Figure IX. Means, standard deviations, Cronbach's alpha, and correlations between main study variables (n = 116).

Path Analysis Results

The model fit between the hypothesized model and the data was acceptable: $\chi^2(129)$ = 193.02; χ^2/df = 1.50; CFI = .92; IFI = .92; RMSEA = .066. In addition, the hypothesized paths between major study variables were significant and in the expected direction (Figure X).

Leadership had a strong positive effect on support structures (.66), which in turn had a strong positive effect on IPC (.82). IPC had a strong positive effect on both team effectiveness (.87) and patient safety (.25). Finally, team effectiveness had a moderate effect on patient safety (.39).

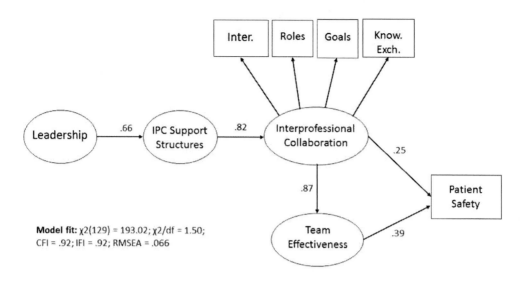

Figure X. Path analysis results.

DISCUSSION

Our findings support past research across a variety of settings that leaders play a key role in facilitating interprofessional collaborative practice (Bainbridge et al. 2010; Goldman, Meuser, Rogers, Lawrie and Reeves 2010; Regan et al. 2015; Stiles et al. 2014). In our study health professionals' perceptions of their leader's contribution to an IPC-friendly work environment by encouraging collaboration and providing access to time, space, and resources (i.e., support structures) were positively associated with IPC suggesting that when such support structures are present higher levels of IPC are likely to occur. Consequently, health care workers' perceptions of IPC were related to higher levels of team effectiveness and patient safety. These findings add to the current knowledge about links between health care leadership, IPC, and patient safety.

Although leaders are thought to play a critical role in shaping health care work environments that support IPC and patient safety, few empirical studies have tested these relationships. The findings of the current study showed that leaders who support IPC by providing access to formalized support structures that facilitate collaboration and communication among team members have a positive effect on IPC. This is in line with previous research showing that leaders who engaged in authentic leadership behaviors and empowered employees by providing them with access to the information, resources, support, and opportunities to accomplish their work facilitated IPC among hospital nurses (Laschinger and Smith 2013; Regan et al. 2015). Formalized support structures that enable IPC to happen can be seen as creating structurally empowering working conditions described in Kanter's (1977, 1993) organizational empowerment theory. These structures create the means to provide information, resources, and support to IPC teams. The strong relationship between leadership and these support structures provides further empirical support for the role of leaders in empowering health care teams for effective IPC.

Organizational support for IPC is an important factor that influences employee attitudes regarding collaboration with other members of health care teams, as well as their ability to actually engage in IPC. Pfaff, Baxter, and Ploeg's (2014) integrative reviews that examined barriers and facilitators of IPC among studies of new graduate nurses found a significant link between formal support from unit leaders and nurses' engagement in IPC. In particular, role modeling and mentorship were important facilitators of IPC. These findings are consistent with Regan et al.'s (2015) study that linked visible and supportive nursing leadership to greater levels of IPC among registered nurses. These studies, along with the results of the current study, show that health care leaders play an important role in promoting IPC in health care settings.

In our study, higher levels of IPC were associated with higher perceptions of patient safety in the workplace, both directly, and indirectly through higher team effectiveness. These findings support the purported links between IPC and patient safety suggested in the various IOM reports (Kohn et al. 1999; Page, 2003). The significant indirect effects of leadership and formal IPC support structures provides empirical support for the importance of empowering leadership as a means for increasing patient safety through collaborative teamwork. To our knowledge this is the first study to make this link empirically.

Limitations

The primary limitation of this study was that it was cross-sectional. A longitudinal design would strengthen the ability to show cause and effect between the model variables. Although the findings provide initial support for the hypothesized model, replication is needed in a larger, more representative sample. Another limitation of the study is that it was conducted in one regional health authority in one Canadian province, which limits the generalizability of the findings.

Finally, although the overall reliability of the scale to measure IPC was good (.79), Cronbach's alpha for each of the four subscales was low. This suggests that addition work on this scale may be desirable in order to strengthen the subscales.

CONCLUSION

Leadership support for IPC is an important factor that influences team effectiveness and patient safety. Creating formalized IPC friendly work structures for health care providers to engage in IPC is one way that leaders can positively influence patient safety within health care organizations.

CASE STUDY

Jonathan Cochrane is a social worker who has been assigned full time to work in the hospital's Rehabilitation Unit. He has always prided himself on his ability to create relationships with other colleagues. He arrives on the unit for his first shift and encounters a very cold reception from the unit clerk and nurse. He tries to allay this first impression to them having a bad day and tries to make conversation with them to learn about the patients on the unit that he needs to assess for placements and other services as part of his role. He finds it very difficult to get the unit clerk to help in identifying patients needing his services. He hears the nurse talk about their bullet interprofessional rounds and ask when these occur. He is informed they are held each weekday at 1 pm in the unit conference room. Jonathan hopes that the rounds today will help him gain access to information about the unit patients and also how he can fit into this rehabilitation team.

During the morning Jonathan continues to approach other staff members to ask if they might need his social work expertise to assist them with their patients and/or their families. Slowly different staff members come to him and discuss how he can assist them with their patients. Jonathan was told at the time of his transfer that the team in this unit was very collaborative. So he prepared to not judge based on his first impressions about the staff and to continue to see a 'place' for himself in their team.

At 1 pm Jonathan shows up in the unit conference room to attend the bullet round meeting. Slowly members of the team arrived and each person comes up to him and introduces themselves. They tell him how wonderful it is to have a full-time social worker assigned to the team. He asks if this role is new in their team. One of the members explains that they had previously been provided with shared social work coverage for their patients but this often led to delays in moving patients forward in their care. The unit manager was instrumental in advocating for this full-time role and finally after many months has been successful. Jonathan is pleased to hear this and considers how the manager had worked to ensure the staff had access to at least one identified structure support, this full-time social work position. He will work to ensure the previous problems with social worker support are no longer a problem for the unit staff. He also feels much more comfortable with the support he is being provided with from other team members. He makes a commitment to himself that he will seek their input about their expectations of him in his role so that all the team members feel they have access to social worker support for their patient care. Jonathan makes a pledge to himself that he will try to spend at least one coffee break with each staff member to learn from them about their roles and also the knowledge, skills, and expertise they can bring to patient care.

Over the next 2-3 months Jonathan becomes an integral team member. He continues to learn from team members while sharing his expertise with them as well. He begins to appreciate how team members work with each other and with their patients to arrive at collective ownership of set goals. There are many opportunities for team members to interact with each other to enhance the care and services their patients receive. It is clear that these team members work interdependently with each other, and he notes the outcome of very satisfied and empowered team members, as well as patients and their families. He also notes the high standards of patient care and patient safety on their unit.

Jonathan also reflects on why this team is so effective and realizes that the unit manager created a quiet but effective set of social norms and workplace culture supportive of IPC. She welcomes staff ideas, listens carefully, and reflects on challenges they present to her. She also recognizes the contributions of individuals and the team in providing excellent care to the patients on their unit.

IMPLICATIONS FOR MANAGEMENT

Promoting a culture of patient safety is at the forefront of nearly all widespread initiatives led by health regions and organizations and is demanded by accreditation bodies. Given the link between leadership and patient safety, it is imperative that formal support structures are integrated throughout the organization to facilitate IPC.

IPC must be incorporated into vision, mission, and/or values statements by executive/senior level managers. Establishing that IPC is an expected practice that is supported by senior management will help to promote the ongoing practice throughout the organization. It is senior management that makes those high-level decisions regarding financial funding and human resource allocation. Recognizing the importance that leadership plays in promoting IPC, team effectiveness, and ultimately patient safety, it would be prudent for senior management to provide adequate funding to hire, mentor, develop, and retain a high functioning leadership team that is committed to the vision, mission, and values of the organization that includes IPC as a key component of its daily business.

Identified competencies for managers at all levels need to be incorporated into performance appraisals/performance management documents so that expectations pertaining to IPC are clearly identified and monitored. Competencies should focus on ensuring that adequate support structures are in place to facilitate IPC. Examples of supports structures include having the necessary policies and/or clinical guidelines to facilitate working with professionals from other disciplines. Focusing on scheduling and having an adequate compliment of workers so that there is time for professionals from various disciplines to meet and discuss patient care is important. Additional support structures include ensuring that unit activity schedules support interprofessional team meetings and/or rounds regularly occurring with the necessary individuals in attendance. Having the actual physical space to meet and discuss patient care is critical. Space is always at a premium in any health care environment; however, room-booking processes may need to be examined so that conference room space is allocated appropriately for IPC activities. Redesigning the physical environment may need to occur and IPC needs to be considered with any new construction.

Aside from support structures, competencies that focus on relationship building and the creation of a conducive environment to IPC should be included in performance appraisals/performance management documents for managers. Relationship building activities can include the promotion of interprofessional education and simulation sessions where professionals exchange knowledge, learn about and understand each other's roles, and recognize the criticality of interdependence and collectively developing and co-owning of patient care planning and goal setting. Creating and fostering an environment where health professionals feel that they are treated as equals, in a respectful work atmosphere in which they can freely share information is not only conductive to IPC and team effectiveness, but promotes interprofessional relationships.

Development of highly effective leadership teams that are able to identify the necessary support structures for IPC, and then facilitate, encourage, and promote IPC in a healthy work environment is not an easy task. It requires much time, effort, and resources. However, if managers are acutely aware of the impact that their leadership actions can have on IPC, team effectiveness, and ultimately patient safety, then the seeding is planted for its realization.

REFERENCES

Bainbridge, L., Nasmith, L., Orchard, C., and Wood, V. (2010). Competencies for interprofessional collaboration. *Journal of Physical Therapy Education, 24*(1), 6–11.

Baker, G. R., Norton, P. G., Flintoft, V., Blais, R., Brown, A., Cox, J., and Tamblyn, R. (2004). The Canadian adverse events study: The incidence of adverse events among hospital patients in Canada. *Canadian Medical Association Journal, 170*(11), 1678–1686. http://dx.doi.org/
10.1503/cmaj.1040498.

Baldwin, D. C., and Daugherty, S. R. (2008). Interprofessional conflict and medical errors: Results of a national multi-specialty survey of hospital residents in the US. *Journal of Interprofessional Care, 22*(6), 573–586. http://dx.doi.org/10.1080/13561820802364740.

Canadian Health Services Research Foundation. (2006). *Teamwork in health care: Promoting effective teamwork in health care in Canada: Policy synthesis and recommendations.* Retrieved from http://www.cfhi-fcass.ca/Migrated/PDF/ResearchReports /Commissioned Research/teamwork-synthesis-report_e.pdf.

Canadian Interprofessional Health Collaborative. (2010). *A national interprofessional competency framework.* Retrieved from http://www.cihc.ca/files/CIHC_IPCompetencies _Feb1210.pdf.

Cheater, F. M., Hearnshaw, H., Baker, R., and Keane, M. (2005). Can a facilitated programme promote effective multidisciplinary audit in secondary care teams? An exploratory trial. *International Journal of Nursing Studies, 42,* 779–791.

Curran, V. (2006). *Collaborative care: Synthesis series on sharing insights.* Ottawa, Canada: Health Canada.

D'Amour, D., Goulet, L., Labadie, J. F., Martín-Rodriguez, L. S., and Pineault, R. (2008). A model and typology of collaboration between professionals in health care organizations. *BMC Health Services Research, 8,* 188. http://dx.doi.org/10.1186/1472-6963-8-188.

David, G., Gunnarsson, C. L., Waters, H. C., Horblyuk, R., and Kaplan, H. S. (2013). Economic measurement of medical errors using a hospital claims database. *Value in Health, 16*(2), 305–310. http://dx.doi.org/10.1016/j.jval.2012.11.010.

Deneckere, S., Euwema, M., Lodewijckx, C., Panella, M., Mutsvari, T., Sermeus, W., and Vanhaecht, K. (2013). Better interprofessional teamwork, higher level of organized care, and lower risk of burnout in acute health care teams using care pathways: A cluster randomized controlled trial. *Medical Care, 51*(1), 99–107. http://dx.doi.org/ 10.1097/MLR.0b013e3182763312.

Etchells, E., Mittmann, N., Koo, M., Baker, M., Krahn, M., Shojania, K., . . . Daneman, N. (2012). *The economics of patient safety in acute care: Technical report.* Retrieved from http://www.patientsafetyinstitute.ca/English/research/commissionedResearch/Economics ofPatientSafety/Documents/Economics%20of%20Patient%20Safety%20- %20Acute%20Care%20-%20Final%20Report.pdf.

Gaboury, I. M., Lapierre, L., Boon, H., and Moher, D. (2011). Interprofessional collaboration within integrative health care clinics through the lens of the relationship-centered care model. *Journal of Interprofessional Care, 25*(2), 124–130. http://dx.doi.org/10.3109/ 13561820.2010.523654.

Goh, S. C., Chan, C., and Kuziemsky, C. (2013). Teamwork, organizational learning, patient safety and job outcomes. *International Journal of Health Care Quality Assurance, 26*(5), 420–432. http://dx.doi.org/10.1108/IJHCQA-05-2011-0032.

Goldman, J., Meuser, J., Rogers, J., Lawrie, L., and Reeves, S. (2010). Interprofessional collaboration in family health teams: An Ontario-based study. *Canadian Family Physician, 56*(10), e368–e374.

Hall, P. (2005). Interprofessional teamwork: Professional cultures as barriers. *Journal of Interprofessional Care, 19*(S1), 188–196.

IBM Corp. (2014a). IBM SPSS Statistics, Version 22.0. Armonk, NY: IBM Corp.

IBM Corp. (2014b). IBM Amos Statistics, Version 22.0. Armonk, NY: IBM Corp.

Kanter, K. M. (1977). *Men and women of the corporation.* New York, NY: Basic Books.

Kanter, K. M. (1993). *Men and women of the corporation* (2nd ed.). New York, NY: Basic Books.

Kohn, L. T., Corrigan, J. M., and Donaldson, M. S. (Eds.). (1999). *To err is human: Building a safer health system.* Washington, DC: National Academy Press.

Laschinger, H. K. S., Read, E., Wilk, P., and Finegan, J. (2014). The influence of nursing unit empowerment and social capital on unit effectiveness and nurse perceptions of patient care quality. *Journal of Nursing Administration, 44*(6), 347–352. http://dx.doi.org/10.1097/ NNA.0000000000000080.

Laschinger, H. K. S., and Smith, L. M. (2013). The influence of authentic leadership and empowerment on new-graduate nurses' perceptions of interprofessional collaboration. *Journal of Nursing Administration, 43*(1), 24–29. http://dx.doi.org/10.1097/ NNA.0 b013e31 82786064.

Lingard, L., Vanstone, M., Durrant, M., Fleming-Carroll, B., Lowe, M., Rashotte, J., Tallett, S. (2012). Conflicting messages: Examining the dynamics of leadership on interprofessional teams. *Academic Medicine, 87*(12), 1762–1767. http://dx.doi.org/ 10.1097/ ACM.0b013e3 18271fc82.

Lown, B. A., and Manning, C. F. (2010). The Schwartz Center rounds: Evaluation of an interdisciplinary approach to enhancing patient-centered communication, teamwork, and provider support. *Academic Medicine, 85*(6), 1073–1081. http://dx.doi.org/10.1097/ACM .0b013e3181dbf741.

Mansour, M. (2009). *Critical care nurses' views on medication administration: An organizational perspective* (Doctoral dissertation). University of Nottingham, England, United Kingdom.

Mazzocco, K., Petitti, D. B., Fong, K. T., Bonacum, D., Brookey, J., Graham, S., and Thomas, E. J. (2009). Surgical team behaviors and patient outcomes. *The American Journal of Surgery, 197*(5), 678–685. http://dx.doi.org/10.1016/j.amjsurg.2008.03.002.

Mitchell, R., Parker, V., Giles, M., and Boyle, B. (2014). The ABC of health care team dynamics: Understanding complex affective, behavioral, and cognitive dynamics in interprofessional teams. *Health Care Management Review, 39*(1), 1–9. http://dx. doi.org/10.1097/ HCM.0b013e3182766504.

Nembhard, I. M., and Edmondson, A. C. (2006). Making it safe: The effects of leader inclusiveness and professional status on psychological safety and improvement efforts in health care teams. *Journal of Organizational Behavior, 27*(7), 941–966. http://dx. doi.org/10.1002/job.413.

Ottawa Hospital. (2007). TOH IPMPC©. *Professional Practice Newsletter, 1*(1), 2.

Page, A. (2003). *Keeping patients safe: Transforming the work environment of nurses.* Washington, DC: National Academies Press.

Parker Oliver, D., Wittenberg-Lyles, E. M., and Day, M. (2007). Measuring interdisciplinary perceptions of collaboration on hospice teams. *American Journal of Hospice and Palliative Medicine, 24*(1), 49–53. http://dx.doi.org/10.1177/1049909106295283.

Pfaff, K., Baxter, P., Jack, S., and Ploeg, J. (2014). An integrative review of the factors influencing new graduate nurse engagement in interprofessional collaboration. *Journal of Advanced Nursing, 70*(1), 4–20. http://dx.doi.org/10.1111/jan.12195.

Poulton, B. C., and West, M. A. (1999). The determinants of effectiveness in primary health care teams. *Journal of Interprofessional Care, 13*(1), 7–18. http://dx.doi.org/10.3109/13561829909025531.

Raab, C. A., Will, S. E. B., Richards, S. L., and O'Mara, E. (2013). The effect of collaboration on obstetric patient safety in three academic facilities. *Journal of Obstetric, Gynecologic, and Neonatal Nursing, 42*(5), 606–616. http://dx.doi.org/10.1111/1552-6909.12234.

Reeves, S., Macmillan, K., and van Soeren, M. (2010). Leadership of interprofessional health and social care teams: A socio-historical analysis. *Journal of Nursing Management, 18*(3), 258–264. http://dx.doi.org/10.1111/j.1365-2834.2010.01077.x.

Regan, S., Laschinger, H. K. S., and Wong, C. A. (2015). The influence of empowerment, authentic leadership, and professional practice environments on nurses' perceived interprofessional collaboration. *Journal of Nursing Management.* Advance online publication. http://dx.doi.org/10.1111/jonm.12288.

Safran, D. G., Miller, W., and Beckman, H. (2006). Organizational dimensions of relationship-centered care. *Journal of General Internal Medicine, 21*(S1), S9–S15. http://dx.doi. org/10.1111/j.1525-1497.2006.00303.x.

Salas, E., DiazGrandos, D., Klien, C., Burke, S., Stagl, K. C., Goodwin, G. F., and Halpin, S. M. (2008). Does team training improve team performance? *Human Factors, 50*(6), 903–933.

San Martín-Rodríguez, L., Beaulieu, M., D'Amour, D., and Ferrada Videla, M. (2005). The determinants of successful collaboration: A review of theoretical and empirical studies. *Journal of Interprofessional Care, 5*(Suppl. 1), 132–147. http://dx.doi.org/10.1080/13561820500082677.

Shortell, S. M., Rousseau, D. M., Gillies, R. R., Devers, K. J., and Simons, T. L. (1991). Organizational assessment in intensive care units (ICUs): Construct development, reliability, and validity of the ICU nurse-physician questionnaire. *Medical Care, 29*(8), 709–726.

Stiles, K. A., Horton-Deutsch, S., and Andrews, C. A. (2014). The nurse's lived experience of becoming an interprofessional leader. *The Journal of Continuing Education in Nursing, 45*(11), 487–495. http://dx.doi.org/10.3928/00220124-20141023-03.

Stutsky, B. J., and Laschinger, H. K. S. (2014). Development and testing of a conceptual framework for interprofessional collaborative practice. *Health and Interprofessional Practice, 2*(2), eP1066. http://dx.doi.org/10.7710/2159-1253.1066.

Temkin-Greener, H., Gross, D., Kunitz, S. J., and Mukamel, D. (2004). Measuring interdisciplinary team performance in a long-term care setting. *Medical Care, 42*(5), 472–481.

World Health Organization. (2006). *Working together for health: The world health report 2006.* Retrieved from http://www.who.int/whr/2006/whr06_en.pdf?ua=1

World Health Organization. (2010). *Framework for action on interprofessional education and collaborative practice* (WHO/HRH/HPN/10.3). Retrieved from http://whqlibdoc.who .int/hq/2010/who_hrh_hpn_10.3_eng.pdf

Zwarenstein, M., Goldman, J., and Reeves, S. (2009). Interprofessional collaboration: Effects of practice-based interventions on professional practice and health care outcomes. *Cochrane Database Systematic Reviews, 3*(3). http://dx.doi.org/10.1002/14651858 .CD000072.pub2

In: Interprofessional Client-Centred Collaborative Practice   ISBN: 978-1-63483-754-5
Editor: Carole Orchard   © 2015 Nova Science Publishers, Inc.

Chapter 8

TRANSFORMATIVE INTERPROFESSIONAL CONTINUING EDUCATION AND PROFESSIONAL DEVELOPMENT TO MEET CLIENT CARE NEEDS: A SYNTHESIS OF BEST PRACTICES

Rosemary Brander[1,2,4], Lesley Bainbridge[3], Janice P. Van Dijk[1] and Margo Paterson[4]

[1]Office of Interprofessional Education and Practice,
Queen's University, Kingston, ON, Canada,
[2]Centre for Studies in Aging and Health, Providence Care, Kingston,
ON, Canada
[3]College of Health Disciplines, Department of Physical Therapy,
The University of British Columbia, P. A. Woodward Instructional Resources Centre,
Vancouver, BC, Canada
[4]School of Rehabilitation Therapy, Queen's University,
Kingston ON, Canada

ABSTRACT

Transformative Interprofessional Continuing Education and Professional Development (ICEPD) takes teaching and learning strategies beyond traditional didactic lecture methods to pedagogical methods designed to match changing health care practices with health professional learning needs. Recommendations for improved health care outcomes include the teaching, learning and application of collaborative practice competencies to better meet individual and population health needs. This chapter highlights a synthesis of best practices for creating effective transformative ICEPD opportunities for health professionals learning about collaborative practice.

Pedagogical strategies encompassing principles for effective interprofessional workplace learning, community learning frameworks, and knowledge-to-practice considerations, are presented. Overall strategies are described, such as the use of blended and interactive learning approaches to address competency-based outcomes, progression from introductory to more complex learning tasks to achieve mastery, and methods for improved knowledge-to-practice transfer for the development of essential and advanced collaborative practices. Measurement strategies targeting desired ICEPD outcomes and the need for the identification of theory to enhance pedagogical choices are emphasized. Investigative change-based strategies and frameworks, such as an ICEPD-Quality Improvement framework to enhance workplace learning, are also reviewed.

It is recognized that a variety of options for learning, through the lived experience, via individual and team feedback related to everyday experiences, and with critical reflection, enhance the mobilization of knowledge for transformational practice change. A case study regarding an application of ICEPD in the workplace directed toward a Patient and Family Centred Care education intervention is provided to enable application of the chapter's main lessons.

INTRODUCTION

Transformative interprofessional continuing education and professional development (ICEPD) takes teaching and learning strategies beyond traditional didactic lecture methods, primarily focused on the individual health professional learner, to pedagogical methods that incorporate processes and contexts to match changing health care practice needs at team, organizational, and community levels (American Association of the Colleges of Nursing and Association of American Medical Colleges 2010; Balmer 2012). These more recent pedagogical strategies demand the use of a blend of learning approaches that address competency-based outcomes (Simmons and Wagner 2009) with a corresponding progression from introductory to more complex learning tasks to achieve mastery (Bainbridge and Wood 2013; D'Eon 2005). Many Canadian universities, preparing health care professionals for practice, focus health care education on six interprofessional competencies (patient/client/family/community-centered care, interprofessional communication, role clarification, team functioning, interprofessional conflict resolution, and collaborative leadership) with the goal of improved collaboration for safety and quality health care outcomes (Canadian Interprofessional Health Collaborative, 2010). We suggest that continuing interprofessional development (CIPD) for the transformation of health care would necessarily build educational strategies based on these competencies.

Blended and interactive learning approaches support a variety of learning styles of health professionals as they develop essential and advanced collaborative practice knowledge, attitudes, and skills with, from, and about each other (Abu-Rish et al. 2012; Centre for the Advancement of Interprofessional Education, 2002; World Health Organization, 2010). Oandasan and Reeves (2005) also suggested pedagogical design for collaborative practice learning requires a mix of delivery formats and approaches, such as face-to-face interactive team process-oriented learning using case studies, simulation, and problem-based learning, and must also address group balance (number of each profession), group mix (eight to 10 participants), and group stability (members stay together). These methods provide options for learning, critical reflection, and feedback related to situations experienced in everyday collaborative practice. This chapter highlights a synthesis of best practices for creating effective transformative CIPD opportunities for health professional learning about collaborative practice and provides a case study to enable application of the chapter's main lessons.

THE LEARNING CONTEXT

Consideration of Learning Context Is Important

Whether in a community context, a hospital, or a private clinic, seamless integration among the education intervention components of transformative CIPD is necessary to effectively prepare and sustain health professionals as collaborative practitioners (Frenk et al. 2010; Kim, Lowe, Srinivasan, Gairy, and Sinclair 2010). The learning setting can be formal, informal, implicit, unintended, opportunistic, or unstructured and self-directed. Formal contexts may involve deliberate learning by engagement in explicitly planned learning opportunities with defined goals, objectives, scheduling, and rehearsing for future events with an educator (Eraut 2004). Traditionally, CIPD is delivered at health professional conferences and academic centers. Embedding CIPD formally or informally within the context of care, often known as workplace learning (WPL), needs further consideration (Brandt, Quake-Rapp, Shanedling, Spannaus-Martin and Martin 2010), as learning that is practice-driven and integrated within the workplace is the new vision for transformative CIPD (Miller, Moore, Stead and Balser 2010). WPL is reported to be cost-effective and to improve individual, team and organizational outcomes (Manley, Titchen, and Hardy 2009). Interprofessional WPL may be key in addressing complexity in health care, as learning is contextual and occurs through interaction in complex environments (Kuipers, Ehrlich and Brownie 2014; Sargeant 2009). Interprofessional WPL may afford "a range of activities and interactions that, by degree, assist learning of different kinds and in different ways" (Billett 2014, p. 208). Learning becomes transformative when the behavior and capability of one person or a team of health professionals evolves in response "to local feedback about the impact of actions" (Fraser and Greenhalgh 2001, p. 800), causing critical reflection about team feedback and resultant change in practice. Through positive transformative learning processes, new knowledge related to how to continuously improve performance is generated. "Learning which builds capability takes place when individuals engage with an uncertain and unfamiliar context in a meaningful way" (Fraser and Greenhalgh 2001, p. 800). Health professionals engaged in these collaborative learning processes can remake and transform their practice as required and with just-in-time responses to local situational needs (Billett 2014).

Nisbet, Lincoln, and Dunn (2013) outline six reasons for the perceived effectiveness of interprofessional WPL: (a) innovation, (b) practice improvement, (c) performance improvement, (d) patient safety, (e) working together, and (f) better patient outcomes. With WPL, the focus is on improving interprofessional practice rather than interprofessional learning (Nisbet et al. 2013). However, it may be difficult to separate working from learning. Nisbet et al. (2013) suggested that for effective WPL "benefits might be gained by making the implicit explicit" (p. 472), such as providing feedback on performance and making learning opportunities more intentional by including interprofessional learning and reflection as part of formal workplace meetings. The learning that occurs *from and through* practice informs *how* to practice (Nisbet et al. 2013). Thus, interprofessional WPL supports transformative learning that occurs through lived experience and critical self-reflection.

LEARNING DELIVERY METHODS

Determining Which Learning Delivery Method(s) to Use Requires Careful Consideration

Designing effective learning opportunities, including which learning delivery method to use, must address the needs of busy health professionals (Kim, Bonk and Oh 2008). In some cases, the use of a community-learning framework may support group learning, particularly group stability in WPL environments. According to Kaplan (n.d.), building an effective blended learning community is based on two core assumptions: (a) the deeper the personal relationships among learners, the richer the collaborative learning experience and (b) relationships among learners are strengthened through structured group interactions using technology before, after, or both before and after a face-to-face learning event.

Two familiar community-learning frameworks, the community of inquiry (CoI; Garrison, Cleveland-Innes, and Vaughan, n.d) and community of practice (CoP; Wenger-Trayner and Wenger-Trayner 2015), are approaches that support interdependence of education and health care as well as interprofessional WPL. By utilizing community-learning frameworks, new knowledge is co-created through "collaborative learning and experiential knowing" (Lawrence 2002, p. 83) using processes of "communication, interdependence, shared responsibility, power, democracy, and conflict" (p. 83). Active learners using a CoI are empowered, that is, they become producers of knowledge, rather than passive consumers of information (Garrison 2007). In the workplace, the use of a CoI framework encourages learners (within and across sites of care) to apply a critical-thinking approach when identifying optimal solutions for a problem (Shields 2003). It is important to note that even though learners come together in pursuit of a common goal, such as developing a collaborative team, the development of a community takes time while relationships grow. "When commitment is high and contributions from all members are valued, communities have the potential to co-create knowledge, make effective decisions, and effect change" (Lawrence 2002, p. 84).

Similar to the CoI framework, the CoP provides a place where people who share a common concern or passion about practice issues can find solutions through regular interactions (Wenger-Trayner and Wenger-Trayner 2015). The learning CoP seeks to develop practice through a variety of methods, including shared problem solving, communicating requests for and responses about information and others' experiences, coordination and consensus, discussing developments, visiting with other members, mapping knowledge, and identifying gaps. Including an interprofessional action project further bridges learning and practice environments within a CoP (Kislov, Harvey, and Walshe 2011). At the organizational, interorganizational, community, and network levels, CoPs can provide a natural, self-perpetuating form of knowledge management and a medium for interprofessional WPL (Kislov et al. 2011).

Supporting an interprofessional learning community network by supplying information technology provides the potential to tightly integrate health professional learning with practice. In fact, the combination of traditional learning with e-learning (i.e., blended learning) can have strategic impact on learning and work processes (Adams et al. 2009; Adams and Morgan 2007; Singh and Reed 2001). Adams et al. (2009) studied the impacts of different levels of blended learning with bank employees. They assessed such impacts as "benefit-cost assessment of the return on learning which measured the tangible and intangible benefits derived from the blended learning study versus the perceived costs to the company" (p. 24). For these bank employees, the return of learning was greater when there was "very tight coupling of personal learning with job performance in relation to the other blended learning strategies" (p. 25). The return of learning was higher for both the individual and the organization when e-learning was blended with face-to-face learning and with collaboration and coaching. This method of delivering education is applicable to health professional learning in the workplace, where both e-learning and face-to-face learning can be made available.

The increased use of new mobile technologies provides opportunities to revisit current learning delivery methods. Blended learning is seen as an increasingly effective method for WPL, as the workplace is where as much as 80 to 90% of learning occurs (Adams and Morgan 2007; Dzakiria, Wahab and Rahman 2012; Kim, Teng, Oh and Cheng 2008; Lee 2010; Lotrecchiano, McDonald, Lyons, Long and Zajicek-Farber 2013). Information technology, when used effectively and efficiently, can integrate education and practice needs through delivery of interprofessional practice-based or point-of-care team learning (American Association of the Colleges of Nursing and Association of American Medical Colleges 2010; Institute of Medicine 2010). In addition, blended learning, when part of a CoP or CoI learning framework, reinforces the role of situated or WPL as a vehicle for directly linking learning and health care outcomes (Miller et al. 2010). This is important, as CoPs, for example, hold the potential to support inter- and intra-collaborative learning, working partnerships, networks, and support interdependence in education.

DESIGNING LEARNING TO IMPROVE KNOWLEDGE

Designing Learning That Improves Knowledge-to-Practice Transfer Is Critical

It is essential that competent collaborative health practitioners and leaders are capable of adapting to changing complex settings (Fraser and Greenhalgh 2001) to meet today's health care challenges (Frenk et al. 2010; World Health Organization 2013). This requires health professionals to learn collaboratively and to effectively apply new learning in order to problem-solve and adapt to evolving practice situations as required. "Millions of dollars are spent every year on continuing education and training, yet some estimate that less than 10% of this expenditure pays off in improved performance at work" (Merriam and Leahy 2005, p. 1). Instructional strategies and theories on how to enhance the transfer of knowledge-to-practice are often missing from the curriculum-design process (Lee 2010; Merriam and Leahy 2005), resulting in an ineffective application of new knowledge, skills, and behaviors (Lee

2010; Merriam, and Leahy, 2005; Wang, Ran, Liao and Yang 2010; Woodall and Hovis 2013). From the literature, there are a number of best-practice pedagogical interventions (e.g., design strategies) to improve knowledge-to-practice transfer. Yamnill and McLean (2001) present three crucial knowledge transfer factors: motivation to transfer, transfer climate, and transfer design.

Motivation to transfer knowledge-to-practice occurs when well-designed education interventions are relevant to learners and support both formal and informal learning that occurs in social workplace settings (Woodall and Hovis 2013). The degree of transfer improves when factors that work for each local learning event are first identified in context and then incorporated into the design of an education program. Teaching the underlying principles about the event (i.e., why it was held, who initiated it, and for what purposes) and explicating the interconnectedness of its various design elements enhances learning transfer (Fraser and Greenhalgh 2001; Lee 2010). Furthermore, aligning interventions with an organization's priorities and culture, customizing for specific local issues and needs (Dudek 2012; Rossett and Frazee 2006); providing self-directed, relevant, tailored experiential learning in multiple environments (personal, professional, formal, informal, and in social and work settings); including reflective opportunities, social interaction, and access to knowledge (Dzakiria et al. 2012; Rabin 2013; Woodall and Hovis 2013), are additional practices that increase knowledge application (Lotrecchiano et al. 2013). When educational interventions are tailored to multiple practice schedules and learning styles, learning transfer is further enhanced. The use of community learning networks (e.g., CoP or CoI) also increases knowledge transfer in the workplace where learning occurs through practice (Ho et al. 2010; Lees and Meyer 2011; Parboosingh, Reed, Palmer, and Bernstein 2011; Urquhart et al. 2013). However, "successful work-based learning needs a sophisticated community of practitioners able to recognize learning opportunities, and who are willing, as well as able, to communicate their professional knowledge" (Spouse 2001, p. 13). Thus, knowledge about the health practitioners and how they practice in an interprofessional team-based workplace environment is key to designing effective and relevant transformative education interventions (Ascher, 2013).

Understanding the knowledge-to-practice *transfer climate*, or contextual factors, and thus the determinants of practice for a particular team or teams of health professionals, guides the design, implementation, and evaluation of tailored educational interventions. Assessment of the determinants of practice at the micro (individual, team) and macro (organizational, community) levels, as well as the barriers or enablers (Flottorp et al. 2013) and the present level of performance gaps (Chevalier 2014), establishes what supports or prevents learning transfer. Flottorp ct al. (2013) created a comprehensive checklist of determinants of practice that focuses on provider behavior (knowledge, skills, attitudes, nature of behavior, capacity to plan change, and self-monitoring), professional interactions (communication, team, and referral processes), incentives and resources (time release, information technology, continuing education, and quality improvement), capacity for organizational change, social, political, and legal factors. The items on the checklist are comparable to the interactional factors outlined in the interprofessional education framework for collaborative, client-centered practice: interpersonal relationships among team members, organizational factors (conditions within the organization) and systemic factors (conditions outside the organization that include social, cultural, professional, and educational systems) (D'Amour and Oandasan 2005; see Figure XI).

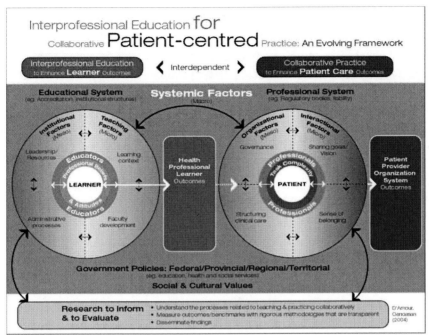

Note. From "Interprofessionality as the Field of Interprofessional Practice and Interprofessional Education: An Emerging Concept," by D. D'Amour and I. Oandasan, 2005, *Journal of Interprofessional Care, 19*(Suppl. 1), p. 11. Copyright 2005 by D'Amour and Oandasan. Reprinted with permission.

Figure XI. Interprofessional education for collaborative patient-centered practice model.

Organizational and team interactional factors, for example, can influence the dynamics of collaboration in the practice setting (San Martín-Rodríguez, Beaulieu, D'Amour and Ferrada-Videla 2005).

Once the local determinants of practice are known, relevant learning *transfer design* strategies, such as the use of scenarios, role-playing activities, and *in situ* simulation (Rosen, Hunt, Pronovost, Federowicz, and Weaver 2012), as well as action projects that address complexity, can assist to further facilitate interprofessional learning adapted to specific care situations (Kuipers et al. 2014). The KT Clearinghouse (2014) lists implementation practice change strategies, including education interventions that promote interactivity such as small groups, continuing professional development, and CoP; linkage and exchange interventions such as academic detailing; feedback interventions such as needs assessments, interviews; electronic interventions such as reminders and eHealth interventions; client-mediated interventions such as health promotion; and organizational interventions such as quality improvement (QI) programs. Leeman, Baernholdt and Sandelowski (2007) linked existing taxonomies with relevant theories to create fourteen implementation practice change strategies organized into five main categories: strategies that (a) increase coordination (e.g., centralizing care management, use of plan-do-study-act cycles); (b) raise awareness (e.g., education provided by external change agents); (c) persuade via interpersonal channels (e.g., interpersonal networks, communication, and use of managers to promote a process change); (d) persuade via reinforcing belief that behavior will lead to desirable results (e.g., data collection and feedback), and (e) increase behavioral control (e.g., reminder systems, changes to work environment such as altering the materials or equipment available, and having a designated change leader). Although originally focused on the nursing profession, strategies that strengthen the health professional's capability to transfer knowledge to the practice setting (Moore, Green, and Gallis 2009) have application to transformative CIPD programs. Further study in this area is needed to determine how to effectively transfer evidence-based knowledge using an interprofessional approach in a variety of contexts for transformative learning; however, some of the best practices cited in this chapter do hold promise for CIPD. To explain this further a case study is provided.

Case Study Regarding Interprofessional Continuing Education and Professional Development in the Workplace

In an exploratory case study, the perspectives of health care providers (HCPs) were explored before, during, immediately after, and 6 months after implementing a well-established interprofessional client and family-centered care (PFCC) education intervention in a local health care organization. The PFCC curriculum is based on the Registered Nurses Association of Ontario (2006) *Best Practice Guideline on Client Centered Care* framework of identifying needs, making decisions, caring and service, and evaluating outcomes. The purpose of the PFCC education intervention was to engage HCPs in enhancing client and family involvement within the organization. A series of eight weekly 2-hour facilitated face-to-face interprofessional group learning sessions, led by trained and experienced course moderators, was held and augmented with pre-reading and written reflections between sessions. To receive PFCC certification, learners completed five assignment conversations with clients and families and participated in at least seven of the eight sessions.

For the research project, the education intervention included participant focus groups and reflections regarding their current knowledge, attitudes, and practices about collaborative care relationships. The researchers proposed that HCPs knowledge, attitudes, and practices related to collaborative care relationships would improve following the interventions. Focus group interviews were held to gain insight associated with the meaning customer service and its relationship to collaborative care and how it may have changed from before, immediately after, and 6 months after the intervention.

Findings

After the intervention, HCP participants expressed a change in their beliefs, in that they now saw clients and families as interdependent knowledge experts and partners. Participants ascribed improved relationships with client and families and to newly adopted practices. These changes were reported up to 6 months after the PFCC education intervention. Many of the emergent themes (communication, respect, shared decision-making, and knowledge) concurred with previously reported determinants for successful collaborations (Orchard, Curran, and Kabene 2005; San Martín-Rodríguez et al. 2005; Suter et al. 2009; World Health Organization 2010) and for improved client safety and error reduction (Howe, Billingham and Walters 2002).

Case study participants questioned the degree to which clients and families understood their rights and the mechanisms to enable their rights to minimize power imbalances between themselves and clients and families. Difficulties in rights enactment were often attributed to existing operational processes within the organization, communication challenges, and historical norms.

Communication, shared-decision making, and mutual respect were identified by the participants as a means to help build relationships and to negotiate power imbalances with clients and families. These were seen as areas for future practice and organizational development to better enable human rights and partnerships within care relationships.

An important finding was that not all HCPs related to 'customer service' as a guide for practice. 'Partners-in-care' was a conceptual framework that was preferred by the participants as it represented a balance of power in relationships. Partners-in-care was suggested as the shared conceptual framework and seen as meaningful by HCP participants seeking to understand the components for successful collaborative health care relationships.

This case study mirrored the four phases that Orchard et al. (2005) considered necessary to create a culture of collaborative practice: participants questioned their own and each other's values and debated the use of language and power (sensitization); explored their roles, decisions, and practices (exploration); collaborated with others who had received the PFCC education (intervention); and shared reflections and new practice implications (evaluation). Peer discussion and inquiry in a safe environment with opportunities to implement new ideas and skills are important for effective practice change (Argyris 1977).

These principles align with the importance of effective interprofessional learning opportunities in the workplace, which include exposure, immersion, and mastery of processes (Grant, Bainbridge and Gilbert 2010). Participants reported that focused discourse, time for independent reflection, and education-in-tandem with real-life workplace practice contributed to attitude and practice changes.

Implications for Practice

This case study is representative of transformational CIPD in the workplace. The educational intervention was directed towards locally identified needs, and comprised a variety of interventions and interactional activities that provided the opportunity for learners to transfer and adapt new learning and skills to the practice environments over time. Formal education in the workplace, with time for reflections during the course and in focus groups, enhanced application of new practices in the workplace.

A community of learning was developed within the organization, which furthered individual practitioner and organizational change towards collaborative practice. Transformative learning and interdependence of education were both achieved with learning and practice aligned and integrated in the workplace.

MEASUREMENT OF IMPACT

Measuring the impact (or impacts) of transformative CIPD program and practice changes on health system performance and population health outcomes is pivotal. Measuring the impact of the transformative education intervention on intermediate (e.g., intervention targets) and longer-term performance outcomes (e.g., patient care and system changes) requires a more rigorous interprofessional education (IPE) research approach that adds to the existing body of evidence (Payler, Meyer, and Humphris 2011; Reeves, Perrier, Goldman, Freeth, and Zwarenstein 2013). In particular, evidence around the IPE elements that support the translation of knowledge into practice (Curran, Sargeant, and Hollett 2007; Zwarenstein and Reeves 2006; Zwarenstein, Goldman, and Reeves 2009) and that will support IPE theory development of new knowledge (Hean, O'Halloran, Craddock, Hammick, and Pitt 2013; Sargeant 2009) is needed. More robust IPE strategies that measure the impact of the education intervention on performance or practice outcomes and health care system-level outcomes will enhance CIPD in the future. However, there is some attention to measuring impact in the literature.

Moore, Green, Jay, Leist, and Maitland (1994), Sargeant et al. (2011), and Balmer (2013) suggest using investigative change-based strategies to capture the complexity of assessing outcomes such as an intersection of curriculum design and knowledge translation (KT) conceptual models. The Canadian Institute for Health Research (2014) defined KT "as a dynamic and iterative process that includes synthesis, dissemination, exchange and ethically-sound application of knowledge to improve the health of Canadians, provide more effective health services and products and strengthen the health care system" ("Knowledge Translation," para. 1). Kitto et al. (2013) also suggest examining the "boundaries and intersections" (p. 82) among continuing education, KT, QI, and client safety domains.

While QI models, such as the Plan-Do-Study-Act cycle, are similar to the KT model, integrating the QI model with CIPD program model is preferred since both focus on team collaboration, context, and the system environment within which activities occur (Sargeant et al. 2011; Wilcock, Janes, and Chambers 2009). Wilcock et al. (2009) emphasized the need to explore "the social context and mutual interdependence of continuous quality improvement, interprofessional working, and interprofessional education" (p. 85) for transformative CIPD programs to be effective in improving performance outcomes. Van Hoof and Meehan (2011) suggested an intervention that focuses on "a prioritized and expanded list of educational outcomes and include three key QI concepts: what interventions work; reasons why interventions work; and what contextual factors may influence the impact of interventions" (p. 207). Key QI concepts such as the reasons why interventions work, as well as the most effective interventions, are measured through learner assessment and program evaluation methods as part of the CIPD–QI framework. The incorporation of more robust IPE strategies into an CIPD–QI framework can build a "new body of evidence that supports approaches and interventions to incorporate IPE and performance within the health care environment" (Balmer 2013, p. 177). Moore et al. (2009) presented a physician learning conceptual framework associated with continuous planning and assessment in continuing medical education focused on higher level outcomes. The framework is organized into an approach that includes information about how physicians learn, useful instructional design strategies, an expanded outcomes framework, and assessment strategies to measure progress of learners and inform educational planning processes. This framework provides additional insights into how best to design and assess continuous interprofessional interventions using an overarching comprehensive transformative CIPD–QI framework.

Investigative change-based strategies when combined with IPE approaches have the potential to provide the needed rigor for outcome measurements. Balmer (2013) suggested that in order to "build and strengthen the integration of CPD [continuing professional development] and quality improvement, linking evidence-based science, needs assessment of performance gaps, and effective educational approaches to reflect the linkage of education and performance improvement" (p. 175) is required. This integrated strategy provides further understanding of what factors, and how these factors (structure and processes), effect knowledge-to-practice and performance outcomes. This understanding strengthens the ways data are collected to support the design of education interventions in order to impact practice change (Canadian Interprofessional Health Collaborative, 2008; Sargeant et al. 2011).

The use of an CIPD–QI frameworks, based on an evidence-informed planned action approach, is also an important knowledge-transfer strategy to promote uptake of evidence by health professionals (Légaré et al. 2011; Van Hoof and Meehan, 2011), researchers and policymakers "who are all essential players in this knowledge enterprise" (Hoffman and Frenk, 2012, p. 5). This strategic approach bridges recommended instructional reforms and development of collaborative partnerships and networks that extend beyond an educational institution's walls to deliver care and measure the impact of that care on client and population health outcomes (Frenk et al. 2010). Furthermore, the combination of continuous improvement methodologies and WPL, particularly in CoP and CoI social learning environments that support continuous learning (Wilcock et al. 2009), demonstrates how a CIPD–QI framework can be embedded in the workplace. This bridging of health professional education and practice illustrates how transformative CIPD education and health professional learning can be "an integral part of the health care system" (Hoffman and Frenk 2012; Moore et al. 1994, p. 18), even when interprofessional health professional teams collaborate across a continuum of care, such as primary care networks (Oelke et al. 2009).

Integrating CIPD and QI within a community-learning framework also provides the infrastructure for further research to build new evidence supporting strategies and activities integrating IPE with performance within health care settings (Balmer 2013). Recent research (Li et al. 2009; Ranmuthugala et al. 2011) suggested that while the learning and knowledge exchange associated with CoPs they also have the potential to support sharing of evidence-based practices and performance outcome data depend on how the CoP is operationalized (Li et al. 2009). It is possible that through workplace integration of CIPD and QI and using supportive technology, health professionals, individually and collaboratively can "gain insight into how to identify problems through undertaking an audit or thoughtful reflection of their practices and then integrating new ideas, methods, and approaches into practice" (Kitto et al. 2013, p. 86). When such knowledge mobilization changes practice behavior, learning is transformational (Fraser and Greenhalgh 2001).

Designing and implementing transformative CIPD programs leading to transformational learning and practice change at individual, organizational, and health system levels is challenging but essential in addressing and solving today's complex health care delivery and population health challenges. Once change is implemented, the next challenges are to sustain, evaluate, and reframe practices as needed in response to the complex and changing landscape of health care requirements.

CONCLUSION

To meet the needs of new health care realities, health professionals must learn together as teams working and leading collaboratively to meet health needs of individuals and communities, locally and globally. To achieve these goals requires a tighter alignment of interprofessional health professional education with desired health care performance outcomes. This is possible through development of transformative CIPD programs that are based on collaboration and competencies; are relevant to the local context; implemented using a variety of interactional activities and delivery methods, within practice settings; and supported by blended information technology and other learning strategies that improve transfer of knowledge through its application to practice. Integrating principles of QI and IPE into a CIPD framework offers renewed opportunities for knowledge mobilization and application and more rigorous investigative possibilities to measure educational impact on learners for local, organizational, system, and population health outcomes.

ACKNOWLEDGMENTS

The Canadian Interprofessional Health Leadership Collaborative (CIHLC) project is a consortium of the five partner Canadian universities (University of British Columbia, University of Toronto, the Northern School of Medicine, Queen's University and Université Laval). The CIHLC project was funded by the Ministry of Health and Long-Term Care and by individual contributions of the partner universities.

The authors would like to take this opportunity to thank a number of people for making this work possible. First, we would like to thank Gijn Biba, Matthew Gertler, Jelena Kundacina, Jane Seltzer, Benita Tam, and Deanna Wu for supporting this project in various ways during their work in the CIHLC Secretariat. Second, we would like to thank the other members of the National Steering Committee Group for their support during this work, both in terms of their invaluable expertise and moral support, namely Sue Berry, Marion Briggs, Serge Dumont, and David Marsh.

REFERENCES

Abu-Rish, E., Kim, S., Choe, L., Varpio, L., Malik, E., White, A. A., . . . Zierler, B. (2012). Current trends in interprofessional education of health sciences students: A literature review. *Journal of Interprofessional Care, 26,* 444–451. http://dx.doi.org/10.3109/13561820.2012.715604.

Adams, J. M., Hanesiak, R., Morgan, G., Owston, R., Lupshenyuk, D., and Mills, L. (2009). *Blended learning for soft skills development: Testing a four-level framework for integrating work and learning to maximize personal practice and job performance* (Technical Report 2009-5). Retrieved from http://irdl.info.yorku.ca/files/2014/01/TechReport2009-5.pdf.

Adams, J., and Morgan, G. (2007). "Second generation" e-learning: Characteristics and design principles for supporting management soft-skills development. *International Journal on E-Learning, 6*, 157–185. Retrieved from http://www.editlib.org/p/19865.

American Association of the Colleges of Nursing, and Association of American Medical Colleges. (2010). *Lifelong learning in medicine and nursing: Final conference report.* Retrieved from http://www.aacn.nche.edu/education-resources/MacyReport.pdf

Argyris, 1977. Cited above.

Ascher, J. (2013). Training transfer: A suggested course of action for local authorities to leverage performance. *Performance Improvement, 52*(5), 36–43. http://dx.doi.org/10.1002/pfi.21348.

Bainbridge, L., and Wood, V. I. (2013). The power of prepositions: A taxonomy for interprofessional education. *Journal of Interprofessional Care, 27*, 131–136. http://dx.doi.org/10.3109/13561820.2012.725231.

Balmer, J. T. (2012). Transforming continuing education across the health professions. *The Journal of Continuing Education in Nursing, 43*, 340–341. http://dx.doi.org/10.3928/00220124-20120725-02.

Balmer, J. T. (2013). The transformation of continuing medical education (CME) in the United States. *Advances in Medical Education and Practice, 4*, 171–182. http://dx.doi.org/10.2147/AMEP.S35087.

Billett, S. R. (2014) Securing intersubjectivity through interprofessional workplace learning experiences. *Journal of Interprofessional Care, 28*, 206–211. http://dx.doi.org/10.3109/13561820.2014.890580.

Brandt, B. F., Quake-Rapp, C., Shanedling, J., Spannaus-Martin, D., and Martin, P. (2010). Blended learning: Emerging best practices in allied health workforce development. *Journal of Allied Health, 39*, e167–e172.

Canadian Institute for Health Research. (2014). *More about knowledge translation at CIHR.* Retrieved from http://www.cihr-irsc.gc.ca/e/39033.html.

Canadian Interprofessional Health Collaborative. (2008). *Program evaluation for interprofessional education: A mapping of evaluation strategies of the 20 IECPCP projects.* Retrieved from http://www.cihc.ca/files/publications/CIHC_EvalMapping StrategiesReport_Sept08_Final.pdf.

Canadian Interprofessional Health Collaborative. (2010). *A national interprofessional competency framework.* Retrieved from http://www.cihc.ca/files/CIHC_IP Competencies_Feb1210r.pdf

Centre for the Advancement of Interprofessional Education. (2002). *Defining interprofessional education.* Retrieved from http://caipe.org.uk/about-us/the-definition-and-principles-of-interprofessional-education/

Charles, G., Bainbridge, L., and Gilbert, J. (2010). The University of British Columbia model of interprofessional education. *Journal of Interprofessional Care, 24*, 9–18. http://dx.doi.org/10.3109/13561820903294549.

Chevalier, R. (2014). Improving workplace performance. *Performance Improvement, 53*(5), 6–19. http://dx.doi.org/10.1002/pfi.21410.

Curran, V., Sargeant, J., and Hollett, A. (2007). Evaluation of an interprofessional continuing professional development initiative in primary health care. *Journal of Continuing Education in Health Professions, 27*, 241–252. http://dx.doi.org/10.1002/chp.144.

D'Amour, D., and Oandasan, I. (2005). Interprofessionality as the field of interprofessional practice and interprofessional education: An emerging concept. *Journal of Interprofessional Care, 19*(Suppl. 1), 8–20. http://dx.doi.org/10.1080/135618205000 81604.

D'Eon, M. (2005). A blueprint for interprofessional learning. *Journal of Interprofessional Care, 19*(Suppl. 1), 49–59. http://dx.doi.org/10.1080/13561820512331350227.

Dudek, J. G. (2012). True learning transfer. *T+D, 66*(7), 80.

Dzakiria, H., Wahab, M. S. D. A., and Rahman, H. D. A. (2012). Action research on blended learning transformative potential in higher education – learners' perspectives. *Business and Management Research, 1*(2), 125–143. http://dx.doi.org/10.5430/bmr.v1n2p125.

Eraut, M. (2004). Informal learning in the workplace. *Studies in Continuing Education, 26*, 247–273. http://dx.doi.org/10.1080/158037042000225245

Flottorp, S. A., Oxman, A. D., Krause, J., Musila, N. R., Wensing, M., Godycki-Cwirko, M., Eccles, M. P. (2013). A checklist for identifying determinants of practice: A systematic review and synthesis of frameworks and taxonomies of factors that prevent or enable improvements in healthcare professional practice. *Implementation Science, 8*, 35. http://dx.doi.org/10.1186/1748-5908-8-35.

Fraser, S. W., and Greenhalgh, T. (2001). Coping with complexity: Educating for capability. *British Medical Journal, 323*, 799–803. http://dx.doi.org/10.1136/bmj.323.7316.799.

Frenk, J., Chen, L., Bhutta, Z. A., Cohen, J., Crisp, N., Evans, T.,. Zurayk, H. (2010). Health professionals for a new century: Transforming education to strengthen health systems in an interdependent world. *The Lancet, 376*, 1923–1958. http://dx.doi.org/10.1016/S0140-6736(10)61854-5.

Garrison, D. R. (2007). Online community of inquiry review: Social, cognitive, and teaching presence issues. *Journal of Asynchronous Learning Networks, 11*(1), 61–72.

Garrison, R., Cleveland-Innes, M., and Vaughan, M. (n.d.). *Community of inquiry (COI).* Retrieved from https://coi.athabascau.ca/

Grant, Bainbridge, and Gilbert. (2010). Cited above.

Hean, S., O'Halloran, C., Craddock, D., Hammick, M., and Pitt, R. (2013). Testing theory in interprofessional education: Social capital as a case study. *Journal of Interprofessional Care, 27*, 10–17. http://dx.doi.org/10.3109/13561820.2012.737381.

Ho, K., Jarvis-Selinger, S., Norman, C. D., Li, L. C., Olatunbosun, T., Cressman, C., and Nguyen, A. (2010). Electronic communities of practice: Guidelines from a project. *Journal of Continuing Education in the Health Professions, 30*, 139–143. http://dx.doi.org/10.1002/chp.20071.

Hoffman, S. J., and Frenk, J. (2012). Producing and translating health system evidence for improved global health. *Journal of Interprofessional Care, 26*, 4–5. http://dx.doi.org/10.3109/13561820.2011.577626.

Howe, Billingham, and Walters. (2002). Cited above.

Institute of Medicine. (2010). *Redesigning continuing education in the health professions.* Washington, DC: National Academies Press.

Kaplan, S. (n.d.). *Strategies for collaborative learning: Building e-learning and blended learning communities.* Retrieved from http://www.icohere.com/Collaborative Learning.htm.

Kim, J., Lowe, M., Srinivasan, V., Gairy, P., and Sinclair, L. (2010). *Enhancing capacity for interprofessional collaboration: A resource to support program planning.* Retrieved from http://www.ahc-cas.ca/repo/en/Confirmed%20resources/IPCEC-Toolkit-Final-Aug-11.pdf.pdf.

Kim, K.-J., Bonk, C. J., and Oh, E. (2008). The present and future state of blended learning in workplace learning settings in the United States. *Performance Improvement, 47*(8), 5–16. http://dx.doi.org/10.1002/pfi.20018.

Kim, K.-J., Teng, Y.-T., Oh, E., and Cheng, J. (2008). *Blended learning trends in workplace learning settings: A multi-national study.* Retrieved from https://wiki-riki.wikispaces.com/file/view/AERA_08_Full_paper.pdf/ 33328621/AERA_08_Full_paper.pdf.

Kislov, R., Harvey, G., and Walshe, K. (2011). Collaborations for leadership in applied health research and care: Lessons from the theory of communities of practice. *Implementation Science, 6,* 64. http://dx.doi.org/10.1186/1748-5908-6-64.

Kitto, S. C., Bell, M., Goldman, J., Peller, J., Silver, I., Sargeant, J., and Reeves, S. (2013). (Mis)perceptions of continuing education: Insights from knowledge translation, quality improvement, and patient safety leaders. *Journal of Continuing Education in the Health Professions, 33,* 81–88. http://dx.doi.org/10.1002/chp.21169.

KT Clearinghouse. (2014). *KT knowledge base: Intervention strategies.* Retrieved from http://ktclearinghouse.ca/knowledgebase/knowledgetoaction/action/interventions/strategies.

Kuipers, P., Ehrlich, C., and Brownie, S. (2014). Responding to health care complexity: Suggestions for integrated and interprofessional workplace learning. *Journal of Interprofessional Care, 28,* 246–248. http://dx.doi.org/10.3109/13561820.2013.821601.

Lawrence, R. L. (2002). A small circle of friends: Cohort groups as learning communities. *New Directions for Adult and Continuing Education, 95,* 83–92. http://dx.doi.org/10.1002/ace.71.

Lee, J. (2010). Design of blended learning for transfer into the workplace. *British Journal of Educational Technology, 41,* 181–198. http://dx.doi.org/10.1111/j.1467-8535.2008.00909.x.

Leeman, J., Baernholdt, M., and Sandelowski, M. (2007). Developing a theory-based taxonomy of methods for implementing change in practice. *Journal of Advanced Nursing, 58,* 191–200. http://dx.doi.org/10.1111/j.1365-2648.2006.04207.x.

Lees, A., and Meyer, E. (2011). Theoretically speaking: Use of a communities of practice framework to describe and evaluate interprofessional education. *Journal of Interprofessional Care, 25,* 84–90. http://dx.doi.org/10.3109/13561820.2010.515429.

Légaré, F., Borduas, F., MacLeod, T., Sketris, I., Campbell, B., and Jacques, A. (2011). Partnerships for knowledge translation and exchange in the context of continuing professional development. *Journal of Continuing Education in the Health Professions, 31,* 181–187. http://dx.doi.org/10.1002/chp.20125.

Li, L. C., Grimshaw, J. M., Nielsen, C., Judd, M., Coyte, P. C., and Graham, I. D. (2009). Use of communities of practice in business and health care sectors: A systematic review. *Implementation Science, 4,* 27. http://dx.doi.org/10.1186/1748-5908-4-27.

Lotrecchiano, G. R., McDonald, P. L., Lyons, L., Long, T., and Zajicek-Farber, M. (2013). Blended learning: Strengths, challenges, and lessons learned in an interprofessional training program. *Maternal Child Health Journal, 17,* 1725–1734. http://dx.doi.org/10.1007/s10995-012-1175-8.

Manley, K., Titchen, A., and Hardy, S. (2009). Work-based learning in the context of contemporary health care education and practice: A concept analysis. *Practice Development in Health Care, 8*, 87–127. http://dx.doi.org/10.1002/pdh.284.

Merriam, S. B., and Leahy, B. (2005). Learning transfer: A review of the research in adult education and training. *PAACE Journal of Lifelong Learning, 14*, 1–24. Retrieved from http://www.iup.edu/assets/0/347/349/4951/4977/10267/F66B135A-DB09-4BA0-8D20-90D751AF39B6.pdf.

Miller, B. M., Moore, D. E., Jr., Stead, W. W., and Balser, J. R. (2010). Beyond Flexner: A new model for continuous learning in the health professions. *Academic Medicine, 85*, 266–272. http://dx.doi.org/10.1097/ACM.0b013e3181c859fb.

Moore, D. E., Jr., Green, J. S., and Gallis, H. A. (2009). Achieving desired results and improved outcomes: Integrating planning and assessment throughout learning activities. *Journal of Continuing Education in the Health Professions, 29*, 1–15. http://dx.doi.org/10.1002/chp.20001.

Moore, D. E., Green, J. S., Jay, S. J., Leist, J. C., and Maitland, F. M. (1994). Creating a new paradigm for CME: Seizing opportunities within the health care revolution. *The Journal of Continuing Education in the Health Professions, 14*, 1–31. http://dx.doi.org/10.1002/chp.4750140102.

Nisbet, G., Lincoln, M., and Dunn, S. (2013). Informal interprofessional learning: An untapped opportunity for learning and change within the workplace. *Journal of Interprofessional Care, 27*, 469–475. http://dx.doi.org/10.3109/13561820.2013.805735.

Oandasan, I., and Reeves, S. (2005). Key elements for interprofessional education. Part 1: The learner, the educator and the learning context. *Journal of Interprofessional Care, 19*(Suppl. 1), 21–38. http://dx.doi.org/10.1080/13561820500083550.

Oelke, N., Cunning, L., Andrews, K., Martin, D., MacKay, A., Kuschminder, K., and Congdon, V. (2009). Organizing care across the continuum: Primary care, specialty services, acute and long-term care. *Health care Quarterly, 13*, 75–79. http://dx.doi.org/10.12927/hcq.2009.21102.

Orchard, C. A., Curran, V., and Kabene, S. (2005). Creating a culture for interdisciplinary collaborative professional practice. *Medical Education Online, 10*, 1–13.

Parboosingh, I. J., Reed, V. A., Palmer, J. C., and Bernstein, H. H. (2011). Enhancing practice improvement by facilitating practitioner interactivity: New roles for providers of continuing medical education. *Journal of Continuing Education in the Health Professions, 31*, 122–127. http://dx.doi.org/10.1002/chp.20116.

Payler, J., Meyer, E., and Humphris, D. (2011). Pedagogy for interprofessional education – what do we know and how can we evaluate it? *Learning in Health and Social Care, 7*, 64–78. http://dx.doi.org/10.1111/j.1473-6861.2008.00175.x.

Rabin, R. (2013). *Blended learning for leadership: The CCL approach* (White Paper). Retrieved from http://www.ccl.org/leadership/pdf/research/BlendedLearning Leadership.pdf.

Ranmuthugala, G., Plumb, J. J., Cunningham, F. C., Georgiou, A., Westbrook, J. I., and Braithwaite, J. (2011). How and why are communities of practice established in the health care sector? A systematic review of the literature. *BMC Health Services Research, 11*(273), 1–16. http://dx.doi.org/10.1186/1472-6963-11-273.

Registered Nursing Association of Ontario. (2006). *Nursing best practice guideline, client centred care supplement* (Rev. Suppl.). Retrieved from http://ltctoolkit.rnao.ca/sites/ltc/files/resources/CCCare/BPStandards/BPG_CCCare_Supplement.pdf.

Reeves, S., Perrier, L., Goldman, J., Freeth, D., and Zwarenstein, M. (2013). Interprofessional education: Effects on professional practice and health care outcomes (update). *Cochrane Database of Systematic Reviews, 3,* CD002213. http://dx.doi.org/10.1002/14651858.CD002213.pub3.

Rosen, M. A., Hunt, E. A., Pronovost, P. J., Federowicz, M. A., and Weaver, S. J. (2012). In situ simulation in continuing education for the health care professions: A systematic review. *Journal of Continuing Education in the Health Professions, 32,* 243–254. http://dx.doi.org/10.1002/chp.21152.

Rossett, A., and Frazee, R. V. (2006). *Blended learning opportunities: American management association special report.* Retrieved from http://www.cedma-europe.org/newsletter%20articles/TrainingOutsourcing/Blended%20Learning%20Opportunities%20-%20AMA%20(Jun%2006).pdf.

San Martín-Rodríguez, L., Beaulieu, M.-D., D'Amour, D., and Ferrada-Videla, M. (2005). The determinants of successful collaboration: A review of theoretical and empirical studies. *Journal of Interprofessional Care, 19*(Suppl. 1), 132–147. http://dx.doi.org/10.1080/13561820500082677.

Sargeant, J. (2009). Theories to aid understanding and implementation of interprofessional education. *Journal of Continuing Education in the Health Professions, 29,* 178–184. http://dx.doi.org/10.1002/chp.20033.

Sargeant, J., Borduas, F., Sales, A., Klein, D., Lynn, B., and Stenerson, H. (2011). CPD and KT: Models used and opportunities for synergy. *Journal of Continuing Education in the Health Professions, 31,* 167–173. http://dx.doi.org/10.1002/chp.20123.

Shields, P. M. (2003). The community of inquiry: Classical pragmatism and public administration. *Faculty Publications-Political Science*, Paper 8. Retrieved from http://ecommons.txstate.edu/cgi/viewcontent.cgi?article=1007andcontext=polsfacp

Simmons, B., and Wagner, S. (2009). Assessment of continuing interprofessional education: Lessons learned. *Journal of Continuing Education in the Health Professions, 29,* 168–171. http://dx.doi.org/10.1002/chp.20031.

Singh, H., and Reed, C. (2001). *A white paper: Achieving success with blended learning.* Retrieved from http://www.leerbeleving.nl/wbts/wbt2014/blend-ce.pdf.

Spouse, J. (2001). Work-based learning in health care environments. *Nurse Education in Practice, 1,* 12–18. http://dx.doi.org/10.1054/nepr.2001.0003.

Suter et al. (2009). Cited above.

Urquhart, R., Cornelissen, E., Lal, S., Colquhoun, H., Klein, G., Richmond, S., and Witteman, H. O. (2013). A community of practice for knowledge translation trainees: An innovative approach for learning and collaboration. *Journal of Continuing Education in the Health Professions, 33,* 274–281. http://dx.doi.org/10.1002/chp.21190.

Van Hoof, T. J., and Meehan, T. P. (2011). Integrating essential components of quality improvement into a new paradigm for continuing education. *Journal of Continuing Education in the Health Professions, 31,* 207–214. http://dx.doi.org/10.1002/chp.20130.

Wang, M., Ran, W., Liao, J., and Yang, S. J. H. (2010). A performance-oriented approach to e-learning in the workplace. *Educational Technology and Society, 13,* 167–179. Retrieved from http://www.ifets.info/journals/13_4/15.pdf.

Wenger-Trayner, E., and Wenger-Trayner, B. (2015). *Communities of practice: A brief introduction*. Retrieved from http://wenger-trayner.com/wp-content/uploads/2015/04/07-Brief-introduction-to-communities-of-practice.pdf.

Wilcock, P. M., Janes, G., and Chambers, A. (2009). Health care improvement and continuing interprofessional education: Continuing interprofessional development to improve patient outcomes. *Journal of Continuing Education in the Health Professions, 29*, 84–90. http://dx.doi.org/10.1002/chp.20016.

Woodall, D., and Hovis, S. (2013). *Eight phases of workplace learning: A framework for designing blended programs* (White Paper). Retrieved from http://www.skillsoft.com/assets/white-papers/eight_phases.pdf.

World Health Organization. (2010). *Framework for action on interprofessional education and collaborative practice*. Retrieved from http://whqlibdoc.who.int/hq/2010/WHO_HRH_HPN_10.3_eng.pdf?ua=1.

World Health Organization. (2013). *Transforming and scaling up health professionals' education and training: World Health Organization guidelines 2013*. Retrieved from http://apps.who.int/iris/bitstream/10665/93635/1/9789241506502_eng.pdf.

Yamnill, S., and McLean, G. N. (2001). Theories supporting transfer of training. *Human Resource Development Quarterly, 12*, 195–208. http://dx.doi.org/10.1002/hrdq.7.

Zwarenstein, M., Goldman, J., and Reeves, S. (2009). Interprofessional collaboration: Effects of practice-based interventions on professional practice and health care outcomes. *Cochrane Database of Systematic Reviews, 3*, CD000072. http://dx.doi.org/10.1002/14651858.CD000072.pub2.

Zwarenstein, M., and Reeves, S. (2006). Knowledge translation and interprofessional collaboration: Where the rubber of evidence-based care hits the road of teamwork. *Journal of Continuing Education in the Health Professions, 26*, 46–54. http://dx.doi.org/10.1002/chp.50.

In: Interprofessional Client-Centred Collaborative Practice
Editor: Carole Orchard

ISBN: 978-1-63483-754-5
© 2015 Nova Science Publishers, Inc.

Chapter 9

THEORY INTO PRACTICE: THE CHALLENGES AND REWARDS OF DEVELOPING AND RUNNING AN INTERPROFESSIONAL HEALTH CLINIC

Daniel O'Brien and Marion Jones
Auckland University of Technology, Auckland,
New Zealand

ABSTRACT

This chapter uses a case study related to an interprofessional team working within an interprofessional health clinic that provides care for clients and interprofessional education and practice experience for health professional students. The focus of the case study is on the application of transformational leadership by the clinic manager who identifies barriers that exist in the clinic operation to meet effective client care. This is explored in the context of structural and process-oriented issues that arose from a client's encounter with the clinic appointment and assessment processes. The chapter then presents the application of transformative leadership in the relation to how clients interact with clinic staff, manage staff capacity, and provide students with interprofessional learning opportunities. Pulling on relevant literature, this chapter reviews both the changes achieved and why these changes were likely realized.

These changes are discussed in the context of the individual, the team, and the institution.

Keywords: Transformational leadership, clinic, collaborative assessment, electronic management system, generic assessment, individual change, team change, institution change

INTRODUCTION

Client-centered, collaborative care needs to involve both clients and health professionals working together to plan appropriate strategies (actions), which are responsive to the client's needs, values, and preferences. These actions take into consideration the cultural, social, and economic contexts within which the client and his or her family live and work. Bechtel and Ness (2010) stress that the five attributes of client-centered care are whole person care, coordination and communication, client support and empowerment, ready access, and autonomy. Client-centered care within an interprofessional clinic needs to consider the preconceived ideas of both health professionals and students. In this way it can capitalize on the opportunities for interprofessional practice so that they learn from, with, and about each other to enable effective collaboration. Clients are best served when health professionals work collaboratively with a shared goal of client-centered care. In order to gain commitment from the staff and students to successfully work collaboratively with each other, barriers need to be broken down. As Gilbert (2005) identified, these barriers can occur at an institutional, team, and individual level.

The following case study exhibits some of these barriers and the changes that need to be made for successful interprofessional learning and practice to take place. Furthermore, it highlights some of the initiatives that can be put in place to facilitate interprofessional learning and collaborative practice in a clinical education setting.

CASE STUDY

Background

Melissa Simonds was recently employed by a university to manage their student health clinic and lead students and staff in embracing interprofessional development practice. The clinic has been running for a number of years with the prime purpose of providing a location for students enrolled in health studies programs to undertake clinical placements. The university provides programs and clinic placements for students in the following health care professions: occupational therapy, physical therapy, psychology, podiatry, speech and language therapy, nursing, and social work. While the different professions in the clinic are all housed within the same building, the student learning and clinical services provided tend to occur in isolation. Each service within the clinic has its own reception, client management systems (appointment keeping, billing, etc.) and medical record systems.

Part of Melissa's job description is to lead the transformation of the clinic from a more traditional, siloed structure to one that is underpinned by an interprofessional approach to clinic management, teaching, and client-centered health care. The university has adapted and adopted the model of interprofessional education developed at the University of British Columbia (UBC; Charles, Bainbridge, and Gilbert, 2010; see Figure XII). The model indicates how, during their studies at the university, students progress from exposure to interprofessional education to immersion in interprofessional learning (IPL) and then on to the integration of client-centered interprofessional collaborative practice (IPCP). Furthermore, the model designates the competencies that the students must achieve to obtain the skills needed to practice in a client-centered interprofessional manner. The role of the university clinic was to provide the practice context to bridge the immersion and integration stages of the model and allow students the opportunity to observe client-centered IPCP and to enact some of these skills themselves within their scope of practice.

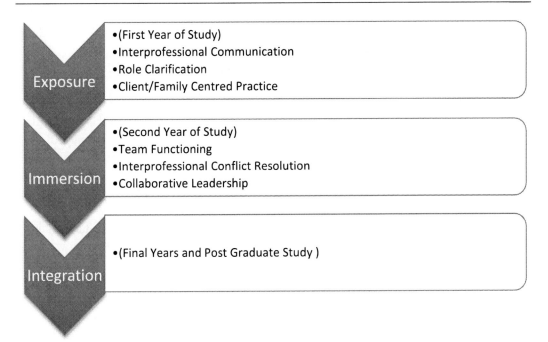

Figure XII. Adaptation of the UBC Model IPE (Charles et al., 2010) adopted by the university.

Melissa has been in the role for five weeks and she now has concerns regarding her ability to transform the clinic to emulate interprofessional client-centered collaborative practice in the manner that her employers desire. She notes that the current clinical services are not client-centered and professionals within the clinic are working in parallel with each other. She feels that many of the processes within the clinic are duplicated. For example, clients coming to the clinic can make appointments with as many as three different reception staff, and can have as many as four separate sets of clinical records (notes).

Melissa has identified potential barriers to the implementation of IPL and practice occurring at institutional, team, and individual levels. These include barriers within the clinic organizational structure and its patient management systems, as well as within the staff's team functioning and their capacity to teach in an interprofessional manner. Furthermore, Melissa feels that there is resistance from staff towards some of her initial suggested changes around systems management improvements (as her professional background is in systems management and not in health care).

Melissa was particularly frustrated by a recent event, when it was discovered that a client (Joan Smith) attended the clinic three times in the space of four days for appointments with different clinicians that all related to a similar condition. She felt that this was not in the best interest of the client and that with some interprofessional communication between the staff and student teams regarding the services provided to the client could have been far more cohesive and client centered, with staff working to achieve a shared goal. Therefore, to get a sense of the client's perspective on interacting with the clinic, Melissa contacted Joan and asked if she would be open to discussing her expectations and experiences while at the clinic. Joan agreed and met Melissa for coffee to discuss her experience. Joan explained that she had been a client of the university clinic for a number of years and really loved the time and attention she received from both students and staff. She also felt that by attending the clinic she was contributing to the students' education, which she liked.

Joan explained that she had rheumatoid arthritis (RA) and, therefore, has a number of different health issues related to this condition. She was pleased that as the clinic had expanded she had been able to see other health professionals without having to go to another clinic. When asked about the three appointments in one week, she explained that the timing made it difficult for her to arrange for transportation, but she was used to seeing different health professionals at different times, saying it was the same as at the hospital. Having lived with RA for 25 years, Joan had spent a lot of time with health care professionals. However, she did agree that had the appointments been timed together it would have saved her husband, who is not a confident driver, three trips to the clinic in one week.

Joan did explain one aspect of the clinic that she found a bit frustrating. She explained that at times a set of notes that had been completed within one service or profession were not always available when she had an appointment with another profession. She said she often felt that she was saying the same things, "telling the same story," over and over again. While she realized that it was important for the students to undertake the interview process with her, she believed if many of them had read her files prior to meeting with her that the sessions would be more productive for all.

Barriers to Interprofessional Leaning and Practice

Based on her observations of the clinic function, discussion with staff and students, and the meeting with Joan, Melissa felt that there were a number of processes that she wanted to change within the university clinic to facilitate an interprofessional approach to learning and practice. She decided for pragmatic reasons to select three key factors that she felt would have the greatest effect on facilitating interprofessional client-centered care. While she had the focus of developing an interprofessional client focused health care service, she felt that she needed to make changes that would affect the culture and systems of the clinic before she focused on more specific service delivery initiatives. Melissa met with all of the clinic staff and three student representatives, she told them Joan's story and then asked them how they believed her experience could be improved. The group chose three factors to focus on: how clients interacted with the clinic staff, staff capacity, and student learning opportunities. The group set goals for streamlining interactions between the clinic (staff and students) and the public (clients and community), implementing strategies to build staff capacity and cohesion, and facilitating more opportunities for interprofessional student learning to occur. The group agreed and a plan was made to implement the recommended changes.

How clients interacted with the clinic. In terms of how the clients interacted with the clinic, all the staff proposed that they centralize the clinic's reception services, meaning that clients attending the clinic would make all appointments and inquiries through a single point of access. This resulted in the reception staff from the different professions being relocated to a single central reception area at the entrance to the clinic. Furthermore, all reception staff developed knowledge and expertise in the different fee structures and booking processes for the different profession-based clinical services. The clinic staff and students proposed a move to an electronic client management system that would allow for the client's clinical records, appointment history, and general health history to all be stored in the same location. This development was staged over time to encompass each of the disciplines located in the clinic. In addition to this Melissa advocated for the development of a single clinic-wide screening and consent form that would be given to all clients who attended the clinic. This proposal was accepted, and a working party was established that included staff and students from each of the professions from the clinic. Each service was asked to provide this group with their existing client screening and consent forms. The group then reviewed the existing forms and collated factors that were duplicated or deemed essential information. A single draft screening and consent form was then designed. This was circulated to staff, students, and clients with the purpose of determining appropriateness and usability. Revisions were made based on the feedback received, and the working group moved to a testing phase across the services. The testing phase resulted in further refinements to the processes of their use, but no further changes were made to the content. This collaborative development resulted in a clinic-wide form being designed and implemented with input from a wide section of stakeholders.

Staff capacity. The next goal was developing the clinical staff's capacity to teach and practice in an interprofessional manner. Melissa sought input from staff and students regarding their views on their current capacity and what might help to enhance their practice and teaching. Firstly, she asked them what their current strengths were. The teaching staff within the clinic commented that they had well-established teams and practices within each profession. However, the staff shared their reluctance to interact outside their designated professions. Furthermore, they commented that there was little opportunity for this interprofessional interaction to occur. Secondly, the clinic had no regular forum for the staff to discuss clinic-wide issues that impacted clinical teaching and service delivery. Melissa proposed the development of a series of both formal and informal opportunities for the clinical staff to interact. She then asked the staff what would work best for them to address these interprofessional gaps. Staff suggested having informal semi-regular shared lunches for clinical and non-clinical clinic staff to get to know each other. The staff then asked for quarterly, formal, continued professional development programs to be provided based on topics associated with interprofessional collaborative teamwork and teaching. Melissa asked what would be important to the staff in shaping these learning sessions, and they commented that these should not be profession specific, to ensure that all who attended would equally value them. They asked that speakers with a specific interest in teaching in the clinical setting be invited to some of the sessions. They also asked that these sessions be facilitated in a manner that forced staff to interact with individuals from outside their own professional group with whom they traditionally worked. Finally, people asked to have monthly all-clinic staff meetings to discuss shared concerns or ideas. Melissa was very supportive of this idea and asked for their input about what day of the month and time these should be held. She then asked who would like to chair the first session. Several staff members volunteered, and the group made a decision that this chairing could rotate around these individuals on a scheduled basis. Establishment of the meetings, the lunches, and the staff development sessions resulted in the staff developing relationships with clinic-based staff whom they did not usually interact with on a regular basis. The monthly clinic-wide service management meetings chaired by staff provided the forum for staff to discuss clinic-wide issues that impacted on their clinical teaching and service delivery. The staff agreed that while it was not expected all staff should attend all meetings, it was expected that each meeting included representation from all professions contained within the clinic, and that notes from the meetings be shared with all staff. Hence, when Melissa changed her leadership approach to one of a true collaborative leader, she was more successful in achieving the changes she sought. The means to achieving these advances was through the use of a shared leadership approach from within the staff.

Student interprofessional learning opportunities. In one of the monthly meetings, the clinic staff addressed the issue of the low number of interprofessional opportunities that students had during their placements within the clinic. This agenda item was put forward following one of their quarterly continuing education sessions focusing on student interprofessional learning. The staff expressed their desire to increase the opportunities that students had to interact and/or learn from, with, and about each other. It was Melissa's hope that by improving the cohesion within the clinical teaching staff across the clinic through informal and formal interprofessional sessions, a desire for the staff to see opportunities to work with staff from different professions than their own would result. Like with the staff interprofessional interactions, she was keen for the interprofessional student learning opportunities to be both formal and informal.

Melissa asked the staff for their ideas around both formal and informal ways the students could gain IPL in their clinic placements. The staff considered the teaching and learning sessions that were facilitated within the clinic and identified upcoming sessions that may have relevance to interprofessional student groups placed within the clinic. They then discussed how to construct these sessions so that they could provide joint teaching and learning opportunities for the students as well. The staff then created a shared teaching plan based on the identified opportunities to guide staff on connecting with each other across their professions and services to facilitate this IPL in student groups. This included steps to reduce the use of uni-professional specific jargon and teaching practices to allow for open communication among the interprofessional student groups. The staff also felt that interprofessional student groups could book combined treatment sessions for selected clients, leading to further informal learning in their placements. Melissa, in collaboration with each service lead and the receptionists, identified criteria that might be used to select these clients. She agreed to bring these criteria for discussion to the next month's clinic staff meeting and to also explore how to test this learning opportunity with a client who would benefit from the combined input of an interprofessional perspective from more than one profession.

Impact of the Implemented Changes

It is not uncommon for staff to be hesitant in embracing the implementation of change processes, and Melissa encountered this with the clinic staff. Initially, it took time for the staff to understand the university's interpretation of interprofessional practice. Many staff members were initially more comfortable working in their familiar multi-disciplinary manner. However, as they tried new approaches, they agreed these beliefs and practices started to change. The changes seemed to become the norm as the clinical staff identified the number of commonalties that they had with the other non-clinical staff and interprofessional staff. Melissa chose to employ a transformational leadership model (Bass 1985) and a collaborative leadership approach to guide the change process within the clinic. Melissa felt that the model was appropriate, as it has been shown to work well in complex uncertain environments and when the followers are challenged and empowered (Bono and Judge 2004).

How clients interacted with the services. Melissa believed that centralizing the clinic's reception and administrative staff and moving to a single electronic-based clinical records system would be relatively simple processes. However, this action highlighted differences between the professions that no one had anticipated. The reception staff had well developed habits that were linked to the preferences and processes of one group of staff and students. They now had to become cognizant of the habits, preferences, and process of all of the clinic service staff and students. Initially, staff felt that centralization had in fact slowed down the client flow processes, but in time this improved.

The second systems-based change that Melissa operationalized was the move to electronic records. This required a reformatting of the clinical spaces so that all staff and students could have access to a computer or a tablet. This also required significant capital expenditure on the part of the university to fund the implementation of both the hardware and the leasing of the software. Another barrier that Melissa had not anticipated was the difficulty that she would experience attempting to identify an electronic client management system (ECMS) that would meet the needs of all of the professions. While many different ECMSs were trialed, most were designed with one profession in mind. This could result in professions, other than the one for which the ECMS was intended, choosing to limit their use of the program.

After piloting a number of different systems, the clinic staff chose a hybrid ECMS that allowed for multiple systems to be combined, meaning that each profession could choose the system that suited their specific needs. All the professional staff worked on a shared generic set of parameters for their care and then each profession's specific ECMS. This was then linked together through a bridging program to the generic record that was used by the reception staff so that both shared and unique client information, assessments, treatments, and outcomes related to identified client shared goals could be combined, functioning like a single client treatment record that was interprofessional and client centered. This hybrid system meant that generic client data could be collected prior to the start of the clinical session. Gathering of client information could also occur on the phone with clinic reception staff when making an appointment, and when the client first arrived at the clinic the receptionist could add greater detail to the client's record. While further profession-specific sections could be added at different appointments or consultation, all staff and students would have immediate access to generic client information and would be able to access additional clinical notes from professions other than their own as needed. This allowed for the specifics of each discipline to be tracked while the links in the system merged to show the collaborative possibilities needed for interprofessional practice. Due to these changes in process, the client's generic information would be collected only once; this positive outcome saved time not only for the client but also for the staff.

Staff capacity. The main facilitator of this change was the instigation of the monthly clinical management meetings, as these allowed the clinical staff to identify many parallel practices (both administrative and clinical) that were occurring in the clinic. These monthly meetings brought the staff together to discuss clinic-wide issues, and in part united the staff over shared challenges and issues. Furthermore, the staff interprofessional development workshops allowed a forum for clinical service-based development to be fostered. Staff had opportunities to discuss potential clinical initiatives that they wanted to develop within the clinic, such as combined clinical services; these opportunities led to some innovative ideas being adopted. The clinic staff became quite stable with little turnover and change. However, one challenge that was identified as the clinic's staff transitioned to working in a more interprofessional manner was the training of new staff when a member left. New staff often required significant education to gain the interprofessional skills that their predecessor had developed. These challenges led to the observation that a staff orientation program to this interprofessional culture was required. The program would give new staff an opportunity to learn about the practices and culture within the clinic, and limit the impact of staff turnover.

Student interprofessional learning opportunities. It was no surprise to Melissa that the students engaged with the IPL activities and practices with great enthusiasm. She felt that many of the students professional socialization was still evolving and these clinic-learning exposures created their capacity for interprofessional practice. While some students found it challenging to work collaboratively with students and staff from other professions, most appreciated opportunities to learn from, with, and about other professions. Students easily came to terms with the notion that to be truly client focused, they needed to be aware of the differences between the client's needs and staff's desire for client's care. Furthermore, students enjoyed interacting with students from other professions, as well as having the opportunity to highlight for their peers how interprofessional practice could be achieved after they had graduated.

CASE STUDY ANALYSIS

A fictitious scenario was presented in the above case study, which outlined many of the barriers and challenges that health care practitioners face when trying to facilitate IPL and practice in a clinical education environment. Melissa used two models to guide the changes within the clinic: Bass's (1985) transformational leadership model as and the UBC model of interprofessional education (Charles et al. 2010). Research has highlighted that these challenges and barriers can exist at an institutional, team, and individual level (Gilbert 2005), and that clear leadership is required to overcome these barriers and challenges. The analysis of the case study explores how these challenges and barriers could be addressed level by level (institutional, team, and individual). It explores the leadership model that Melissa engaged in to facilitate the changes, and finally explores the student's role in the case study.

Leadership is needed in any change process. The transformational leadership model fits well into the environment of IPCP, as it is by its nature a collaborative process (Bass 1985). Furthermore, Bass's (1985) model is underpinned by the notion that transformational leadership encompasses intellectual stimulation, individual consideration, inspirational motivation, and idealized influence. The staff developed motivation to change through the role modeling and staff development along with a common vision and recognizing the challenges in the change occurring. Working together over the time of the change, from working in parallel to working together with each other, provided staff with the motivation to do more in learning from each other to develop the best plan of care for the client (see Figure XIII).

Institutional. At an institutional level, three factors presented in this case study acted as barriers to the implementation of interprofessional education and collaborative practice. These included the clinic staff management structure, the administrative structure, and funding. It may be argued that if health care practitioners have the necessary skill set to practice in a collaborative interprofessional client-centered manner that they should be able to undertake this practice in any environment. However, institutional environments, cultures, and practices can often impose barriers to effective client-centered and/or interprofessional practice (Gilbert 2005).

Level	Barriers	Solutions
Institutional	The lack of a clear mandate Clinic management structure Clinic systems Funding	Establishment of a faculty mandate Establishment of a monthly clinic-wide staff meeting Centralized clinic reception Electronic notes Clinic-wide client screening form Re-centralizing of services
Team	Staff capacity and understanding of IPE and IPCP Limited shared purpose Limited opportunities for students to engage in IPE and IPCP	Collaboration with staff to develop informal meetings, continued staff development, monthly staff meetings Team development
Individual	Staff beliefs and attitudes Parallel working Discipline boundaries	Opportunities for staff to collaborate led to shifting attitudes and beliefs Breakdown of perceived discipline boundaries

Note IPE= Interprofessional Education; IPCP = Interprofessional Collaborative Practice.

Figure XIII. An overview of the identified barriers at each level and how they were mitigated.

This is especially the case if the systems, culture, or environment makes it easier for health care professionals to work in a uni-professional or multi-professional manner. This is often the situation in health care systems that are already strained and understaffed. Health professional educators often argue that interprofessional practice takes more time and is less time efficient (Gilbert 2005). These interprofessional tensions are compounded when health professional students are included, as this requires that staff also provide clinical education. The health professional practitioner's focus is now divided between meeting the needs of the client, the service (institution), and students.

With all these tensions in place, it is essential that barriers to collaborative interprofessional client-centered practice at an institutional level be removed or mitigated. Initially, within the clinic staff appeared to lack knowledge and appreciation of each other's roles and responsibilities, so parallel working was the norm. With Melissa working with the team to develop a commitment to collaborative practice and focus on client-centered interprofessional practice, staff developed the willingness to work together and share responsibility for the client. Overtime, this developed confidence, trust, and respect for each other's work.

The administrative structure was changed to be in line with a common assessment process, and the interprofessional meetings helped support a forum for moving in the direction for collaboration. By working more efficiently and effectively the funding issue became less of a problem, as savings were achieved by the decreased staff turnover and centralized appointments. These savings meant that Melissa could reallocate funds to cover the additional costs.

Having an institutional mandate for transparency in meeting performance indicators from the senior executive team provides a momentum to support clinic changes. The commitment of clinic staff and the university faculty who support the services and student placements also helped make the changes successful.

Systems were put in place that overcame these barriers and challenges over time. The major change for the clinic staff and its clients was the collaborative assessment tool, which is now consistently used. Introducing a new culture, as this case study demonstrated, must always include an institutional focus initially, along with the team and individual impact considerations.

Team. The following barriers are commonly cited to IPCP at a team level: no shared vision or purpose, limited understanding of IPCP and IPL, no team building, apathy or conflict within the team, and a hierarchical team structure (Gilbert, 2005). Within the case study barriers to IPCP and IPL occurred at a team level and included both the lack of a shared vision or purpose within the team and limited understanding of IPCP and IPL. The service teams that had developed within the clinic had been profession-specific teams. Therefore, staff were offered little opportunity for interprofessional team building outside of these existing groups. Additionally any goals, vision, or purpose had been established on a profession-specific basis. Factors identified that can facilitate development of interprofessional team working include collaborative leadership, role clarification, and interprofessional communication (Charles et al. 2010). In this case study, the clinic manager employed a collaborative leadership approach, underpinned by Bass's (1985) transformational leadership model, to facilitate change within the clinic staff.

By involving the staff, students, and clients, Melissa empowered stakeholders to assist in the changes within the clinic and demonstrated the motivation and intellectual stimulation inherent in the model used. Furthermore, by instituting regular clinic meetings and quarterly staff development sessions, the clinic manager facilitated interprofessional communication and role clarification. This led to the building of an interprofessional collaborative clinic team that was no longer bounded by single professions, thereby leading to the development of a shared vision and a better understanding of IPCP as staff integrated their learning into practice.

Individual. Research has indicated that individuals' beliefs, attitudes and ignorance can form significant barriers to IPCP (Curran, Deacon, and Fleet, 2005; Hall, 2005). Discipline focus can often override IPCP. Staff may lack trust and knowledge as well as incentives for IPCP, and professionals can become accustomed to uni-professional role or multidisciplinary practices (Gilbert 2005). Similar to the barriers present at a team level, within this case study Melissa and her staff employed strategies with the purpose of overcoming individuals' profession-specific beliefs and attitudes.

By giving clinic staff opportunities to interact both formally and informally, Melissa facilitated development of relationships that spanned professions. These relationships, if nurtured, will allow for diffusion of knowledge and understanding across professions and potentially lead to development of "trust-based relationships" (Hughes and McCann, 2003). These "trust-based relationships" are essential for effective interprofessional practice, collaborative leadership, and interprofessional communication (Hughes and McCann 2003; Pullon 2008). Change can be scary for many professionals in any situation; Melissa attempted to mitigate this by engaging staff, students, and clients in the change process. In doing so, she ensured that the changes were staff, student, and client centered.

This practice is essential for effective transformational leadership. Students' role in the case study. What is quite clear in the case study is that students did not form a barrier to IPL and collaborative practice (Hoffman, Rosenfield, Gilbert, and Oandasan 2008). Exploration and evaluation of student IPL experiences shows that students are typically keen to engage in such programs (Solomon et al. 2010) and appreciate opportunities to learn from, with, and about other health care students (O'Brien, McCallin, and Bassett 2013). However, engaging students in the design, implementation, and evaluation of both IPL and collaborative learning opportunities will surely improve their effectiveness and perceived value of this practice.

CONCLUSION

Reiterating Bechtel and Ness (2010), the five attributes of client-centered care are critical in the consideration of the clinic development. The whole-person care and coordination and communication among and between staff, students, and clients have been more visible as a result of the changes. This appears to have empowered the staff and students. Additionally, client support and ready access to interprofessional care has not only provided further autonomy for clients but also for health professionals, which has been preserved through their interprofessional working. Moving IPCP systems forward can only result when interprofessional interactions are facilitated within clinic or by practice staff. Professional development is critical for this to happen to ensure all participants in practice understand and work within an interprofessional framework supporting learning from, with, and about each other. This is where Charles et al.'s (2010) UBC model provided the key steps for education and practice development appropriate for students' stage of learning in the discipline curriculum. The model locates the point at which the integration and progression of knowledge, practice, and learning occurs. In this case study, team development was seen as essential to support a change from parallel working within each service to IPCP throughout the clinic. The next steps needed are development of further interprofessional work supporting career and succession planning. Bass's (1985) transformational leadership provided Melissa with the model that encompassed tools needed to lead the change process.

REFERENCES

Bass, B. M. (1985). *Leadership and performance beyond expectations*. New York, NY: Free Press.

Bechtel, C., and Ness, D. L. (2010). If you can build it, will they come? Designing truly patient-centered health care. *Health Affairs, 29,* 914–920. http://dx.doi.org/10.1377/hlthaff.2010.0305.

Bono, J. E., and Judge, T. A. (2004). Personality and transformational and transactional leadership: A meta-analysis. *Journal of Applied Psychology, 89,* 901–910. http://dx.doi.org/10.1037/0021-9010.89.5.901.

Charles, G., Bainbridge, L., and Gilbert, J. (2010). The University of British Columbia model of interprofessional education. *Journal of Interprofessional Care, 24,* 9–18. http://dx.doi.org/10.3109/13561820903294549.

Curran, V. R., Deacon, D. R., and Fleet, L. (2005). Academic administrators' attitudes towards interprofessional education in Canadian schools of health professional education.

Journal of Interprofessional Care, 19(Suppl. 1), 76–86. http://dx.doi.org/ 10.1080/13561820500081802.

Gilbert, J. H. V. (2005). Interprofessional learning and higher education structural barriers. *Journal of Interprofessional Care, 19*(Suppl. 1), 87–106. http://dx.doi.org/ 10.1080/13561820500067132.

Hall, P. (2005). Interprofessional teamwork: Professional cultures as barriers. *Journal of Interprofessional Care, 19*(Suppl. 1), 188–196. http://dx.doi.org/10.1080/ 13561820500081745.

Hoffman, S. J., Rosenfield, D., Gilbert, J. H. V., and Oandasan, I. F. (2008). Student leadership in interprofessional education: Benefits, challenges and implications for educators, researchers and policymakers. *Medical Education, 42*, 654–661. http://dx.doi.org/10.1111/j.1365-2923.2008.03042.x.

Hughes, C. M., and McCann, S. (2003). Perceived interprofessional barriers between community pharmacists and general practitioners: A qualitative assessment. *The British Journal of General Practice, 53*, 600–606.

O'Brien, D., McCallin, A., and Bassett, S. (2013). Student perceptions of an interprofessional clinical experience at a university clinic. *New Zealand Journal of Physiotherapy, 41*(3), 81–89.

Pullon, S. (2008). Competence, respect and trust: Key features of successful interprofessional nurse-doctor relationships. *Journal of Interprofessional Care, 22*, 133–147. http://dx.doi.org/10.1080/13561820701795069.

Solomon, P., Baptiste, S., Hall, P., Luke, R., Orchard, C., Rukholm, E., Damiani-Taraba, G. (2010). Students' perceptions of interprofessional learning through facilitated online learning modules. *Medical Teacher, 32*, e391–e398. http://dx.doi.org/10.3109/ 0142159X.2010.495760.

In: Interprofessional Client-Centred Collaborative Practice   ISBN: 978-1-63483-754-5
Editor: Carole Orchard   © 2015 Nova Science Publishers, Inc.

Chapter 10

MOVING FROM ATHEORETICAL TO THEORETICAL APPROACHES TO INTERPROFESSIONAL CLIENT-CENTERED COLLABORATIVE PRACTICE

Sarah Hean[1], Shelley Doucet[2], Lesley Bainbridge[3], Valerie Ball[3],
Liz Anderson[4], Clive Baldwin[8], Chris Green[9], Richard Pitt[10],
Stefanus Snyman[11], Mattie Schmidtt[5], Phil Clark[6],
John Gilbert[3] and Ivy Oandasan[7]

[1]University of Bournemouth, Bournemouth, UK
[2]University of New Brunswick St. Johns, NB, Canada
[3]University of British Columbia, Vancouver, BC, Canada
[4]University of Leicester, Leicester, UK
[5]Rochester University, Rochester, NY, US
[6]University of Rhode Island, Kingstone, Rhode Island, US
[7]University of Toronto, Toronto, ON, Canada
[8]St. Thomas University, Fredericton, NB, Canada
[9]University of Essex, UK
[10]University of Nottingham, Nottingham, UK
[11]University of Stellenbosch, South Africa

ABSTRACT

In response to the importance of theory in the development of interprofessional client-centered education and practice (IPCEP), a novel workshop model, promoting the development of theoretical approaches to interprofessional client-centered collaborative practice in its participants, has been developed. The theoretical underpinnings and development of this workshop model are described in this chapter, which include the concept of coproduction and the use of narrative as a boundary-crossing object between theorist and practitioner. Resources used and means of delivering the workshop are described, in parallel with the first iteration of atheoretical competency framework, proposed to underpin the development of positive attitudes, skills, and knowledge of appropriate theory in this field and to enable practitioners to articulate, defend, reflect, and improve their practice in interprofessional client-centered collaborative practice.

Keywords: Workshop model, theory, co-creation, transformation of knowledge, use of narrative, theorist and practitioner, enabling, improvement of practice

INTRODUCTION

In this chapter we revisit the importance of theory in the development of IPCEP. We focus specifically on the theoretical underpinnings and the development of a workshop model aimed at moving practitioners from atheoretical to theoretical collaborative practice. Theory is a set of propositions or hypotheses linked by a rational argument (Jary and Jary 1995). It has a central role for us as practitioners, guiding us when we engage with new health and social care practices. Theory can help us articulate, reflect, and potentially reinterpret our existing and habitual practices. As humans, we are natural theorists, using lay theory to anticipate and rationalize our everyday activity. However, as practitioners we often have neither the time nor are we in the habit of stopping to reflect on and make explicit our theoretical foundations: the mechanisms by which our actions are expected to have an effect (Pawson and Tilley 1997). We may have developed negative attitudes to theory, seeing it as the antithesis of constructive practice activity. Alternatively, we may see popular theories used in the IPCEP world as either overly reductionist or incomprehensible and complicated.

As a result, we miss an opportunity to use theory as a tool to help us to engage in second-order reflection in which we can stand outside ourselves looking in on our daily practices with a critical eye (Wackerhausen 2009), as an informed guide for our future actions to help find solutions, or to be held accountable for our actions.

In fact, it has been argued that a failure to clearly articulate the theory behind what we are doing is, at worst, tantamount to malpractice (Eraut 2003).

Interprofessional education (IPE), in the past, has been lamented as lacking an evidence-based theoretical foundation (Barr, Koppel, Reeves, Hammick and Freeth 2005, Clark 2006, Craddock, O'Halloran, McPherson, Hean and Hammick 2013, Freeth Hammick, Koppel, Reeves and Barr 2002, Hean, Hammick et al. 2009). Clifton, Dale and Bradshaw (2007), for example, found that only 50% of the studies they selected in a review of the IPE literature had mentioned explicitly the use of an educational or practice theory. However, over the past 10 years, the IPCEP community has started to move from atheoretical to theoretical approaches to interprofessional client-centered collaborative practice. This shift has counteracted the shortfall of IPCEP theory through searching other disciplines for theories that may have utility in the field (Hean, Craddock and Hammick 2012, Helme, Jones and Colyer 2005, Kitto, Chesters, Thistlethwaite and Reeves 2011). The development of the IN-2-THEORY community of practice and the special edition on theory in the *Journal of Interprofessional Care* (Reeves 2013) reflect the commitment to this area.

IN-2-THEORY As an International Community of Practice

IN-2-THEORY is an international community of practice (CoP) that aims to build theoretical rigor in IPCEP. The CoP developed from a series of workshops funded by the United Kingdom Economics and Social Research Council. This brought together individuals interested in theory within the IPCEP field to work together to raise the profile of theory within IPE, research, policy, and collaborative practice (Hean et al. 2013). These workshops developed strong working relationships among international colleagues, and these affiliations led to development of the IN-2-THEORY community (IN-2-THEORY 2010).

Since its inception in 2010, members of IN-2-THEORY have published together on theoretical issues, successfully competed for research funds, delivered workshops on the use of theory in curriculum development, and are currently engaged in a scoping review of theory (Hean, O'Halloran et al. 2012). These collaborations are gaining impetus and the CoP membership is growing. The ongoing activities have developed relationships required to collaborate better in the future. We have had opportunities to learn together about different theories and how these may be applied (Hean et al. 2013).

The increased interest in theory has resulted in an abundance of theories on offer to interprofessional clinicians, curriculum developers, and researchers. The number and variety of theories has raised concerns that these may muddy, rather than clarify, the ways in which theory can contribute to the development of IPCEP.

There is some appeal in identifying a single theoretical approach for consistency and clarity. The Institute of Medicine (2015), for example, has brought together a useful conceptual model capturing the many dimensions of IPE, with the aim of achieving some consistency in terminology and links between health and education systems.

However, theories that underpin relationships between these dimensions are less easily synthesized into a single entity. In fact, the identification of a single theory, capable of explaining all dimensions of IPE or IPCEP, remains elusive and perhaps undesirable in such a complex field, where different groups of learners meet for a variety of purposes and at different stages of their professional development (Barr et al. 2005, Hean, Hammick et al. 2009). A toolbox approach to theory application may be more useful (Hean, Hammick et al., 2009). Theories are drawn from a number of academic disciplines, including sociology, psychology, education, and management. Box 4 provides an illustration of some of the tools available. The key is to select a theory for its ability to articulate or improve the understanding of a specific dimension of IPCEP in a particular context.

Prioritization of a single theory is again inappropriate, as individual theory users have differing preferences and familiarity with theories. Preference may be dependent on one's own unique professional and academic histories. Theories are not mutually exclusive and may overlap with a number of existing frameworks (Hean, Hammick et al. 2009).

It can also be argued that what is now more important in the IPCEP field is a focus on the use of theory, rather than the identification of a single most relevant theory. We, therefore, devote the rest of this chapter to a discussion of theoretical competence and development of a workshop model designed to advance these competencies. This workshop model was developed as a result of the joint activity of In-2-THEORY members.

THE WORKSHOP MODEL

The workshop model was developed from the initial set of workshops funded by both the United Kingdom Economics and Social Research Council and the Canadian Institutes of Health Research between the years 2007 and 2014. The model has been piloted and developed through a series of iterative presentations and workshops at Collaborating across Borders IV and Altogether Better Health VII conferences from 2010 to 2015. The workshop model has also been trialed with doctoral students in a Norwegian national doctoral research-training program (PROFRES 2014).

Workshop Aim

The aim of the workshops was to encourage IPCEP practitioners to use theory to reflect critically on their practice and problem solve within their real-life experiences. These workshops provide a forum for participants to explore how theory can be best applied and practically useful in addressing challenges in interprofessional education and collaborative practice.

Participants are expected to improve their understanding of how theory relates to their practical experiences, be able to identify some relevant theories applicable to this learning, and applicable to this learning, and apply relevant theory to generate innovative solutions to practice problems.

Workshop Participants

Participants are described as practitioners, but in this chapter we will use practitioners to refer to a wider range of stakeholders (clinical practitioners, educators, as well as researchers), as all of these roles require an engagement with theory to underpin their practice activity. For example, for clinical practitioners, theory might underpin the strategies they employ to work with other professionals in their work team or transfer information from one organization to another. For educators, theories on how learning takes place can underpin the interprofessional learning activity. For researchers, theory could underpin variables selected for measurement in the evaluation of an interprofessional collaboration or IPE program.

Co-Creation Process

These workshops are underpinned by the concept of co-creation. Co-creation is the generation of outputs that have added public value and are the result of positive joint activity between two or more actors (Alford, 2009). There is an element of interdependence in co-creation relationships, and the added value should outweigh resources (time, human, financial, etc.) required to engage in the co-creation process (Alford 2009).

The theorist and the practitioner are the two actors brought together in the workshop to co-create new solutions to practice-based problems in IPE or collaborative practice. Their knowledge is interdependent, as the theorist cannot develop and test her or his theory without a practice context in which to test the theory. Practitioners need theory as a tool to guide and rationalize their actions.

Carlile (2004) describes the co-creation process in terms of knowledge passing across three boundaries. First, knowledge must transfer between the theorist and practitioner. Second, transfer of knowledge alone, didactically, is insufficient, as knowledge must then be translated into a commonly understood language. Finally, transformation of knowledge is required.

Transformation of knowledge occurs when political differences are put aside and the theorists' knowledge merges with practitioners' knowledge to form a new perspective on the practice problem at hand. This transformation is reminiscent of Mezirow's (1997) description of transformational learning. For Bernstein (1971, see also Hammick 1998), crossing this final barrier allows for the two very different domains of practitioner and theorist knowledge to overlap to form a new and interdisciplinary region of knowledge where innovative solutions, not attainable by either party alone, are found.

These workshops attempt to mirror this transfer, translation, transformation process, by bringing both parties together to exchange knowledge and co-create a new practice context narrative seen through a theoretical lens (see Figure XIV). The workshops also seek to impart theoretical competence to participants so they will be able to transfer their learning from the workshop back to their own practice. The workshops achieve this in four main phases:

◆ Presentation of theorists' knowledge (transfer and translation).
◆ Presentation of practitioners' knowledge (transfer and translation).
◆ Co-creation of innovative solutions to practice problems using theory as a tool (translation and transformation).
◆ Presentation of theoretical underpinnings of workshop (highlighting theoretical quality and competence).

Practitioners' Knowledge: The Use of Narrative

A narrative or story is the way we as humans arrange our experiences and make meaning of them (Fisher 1987). Humans are natural storytellers. The narrative is both a form of knowledge (the knowledge of the practitioner), as well as a boundary object (Carlile 2004) that facilitates translation of the practitioner's professional knowledge into common knowledge so that it can be understood by the theorist. We have used two approaches to create this narrative. The first involves getting practitioners to tell their story to the group for exploration.

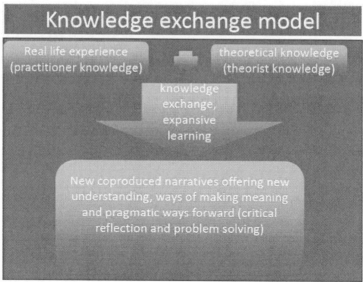

Note: From "Developing Theoretical Rigour in Interprofessional Education" by S. Hean in E. Willumsen, A. Ødegård and T. Sirnes (Eds.), *Collaboration: Theory and Practice*, 2014, Oslo, Norway: Publisher. Copyright 2014 by S. Hean. Reprinted with permission.

Figure XIV. Overlap of practitioner and theorist knowledge to encourage critical reflection and problem solving.

Box 1. Illustration of Questions Used to Extract a Relevant Narrative Pre-Workshop or During Workshop Proceedings

- Tell me about your experience of working in an interprofessional team?
- Think of a specific event in which team working may or may not have worked well.How were things before this event?
- Describe what happened?
- Tell me about the people involved?
- How did this make you feel?
- What values of yours are realized in this story?
- Choose another professional working in the team. How do you think they might have told the story of this event?
- How might we retell the story differently for a different outcome?
- Come up with two things you might do differently and why?

Box 1 illustrates some of the prompts used to extract a rich story. The advantage of participants developing their own narrative is the direct relevance of the story to their own experience, making them more likely to engage with a transformation process. The disadvantage is that it is logistically difficult to get around to everyone's story in a workshop group, and the story of the most dominant individual may take precedence.

Further, stories are often personal, revealing potentially vulnerable elements of an individual storyteller's character or history. The interpretation of the story through theory by fellow participants exposes the participant to potentially damaging reflections on the story and its meaning. The second approach, which overcomes some of the above disadvantages, involves providing participants with a range of pre-prepared stories representing experiences of different stakeholders in IPCEP. Participants, in small group work, must choose one narrative for further analysis. The story chosen may not always be relevant for all participants, however, so it is worth having a range of stories available for theory application (experiences of the IPE curriculum developer, clinician, facilitator or preceptor, student, patient, or researcher) and allowing participants to choose which is relevant to them.

Theorists Knowledge

Transfer of theorist knowledge happens through a brief 3-minute sell of various theories, poster presentations, or reading of summary sheets developed and presented by facilitators in each workshop. Participants are provided with some relevant theories that have potential application to the provided narratives. Participants then discuss the theories with a facilitator in small group work for clarification as required. These facilitators are individuals who are part of the workshop guidance team who have general or particular theoretical expertise, although often they will also have a dual identity as practitioners. As such, they also act as boundary objects (Walker and Nocon 2007), individuals able to transcend interdisciplinary boundaries to translate theoretical knowledge into a format understandable by practitioners.

Theory is presented as a tool to help the practitioner, alongside the theorist, reflect on the practice problem or story. The theory enables workshop participants to make alternative meanings of the same experience or story and potentially alter its trajectory. Box 2 illustrates this by showing that two different theories can provide very different interpretations of the same story. Both theories need to be tested.

Box 2. Narrative Being Interpreted Differently Through Two Separate Theories

---

Story: (courtesy of Clive Baldwin), St Thomas University, Canada
A woman comes into a hospital with a sick child.
The patient notes indicate this is the fourth admission.
The diagnosis of the child's condition is unclear.

What happened next?

Theory 1:
Proposition 1: The child has a complex condition.
Proposition 2: The health professional has not yet identified the condition accurately.

Response: We need to run tests so that the health professional can identify and treat the condition.

Theory 2:
Proposition 1: the mother suffers from Munchausen by Proxy.
Proposition 2: The child is ill because of the mother's condition.

Response: Engage social services to support family, mother and child.

The problem with the example in Box 2, of course, is that one of the stories is essentially true and the other is not — they are mutually exclusive. This is not the case in the application of theory within IPCEP, however, as theories are essentially different lenses bringing into focus different elements of the same problem. One approach is not necessarily more or less useful than the other.

Participants are presented with theories from sociology, psychology, organizational theory, and education, representing micro and macro levels of analysis. Box 3 summarizes some of the theories used in previous workshops. The selection of theories is based largely on their current application to the IPCEP world, but also on the familiarity of facilitators with these particular frameworks. The list, of course, is not exhaustive, so participants are encouraged to use any theory they are familiar with if they see that it has application, as long as they are able to clearly articulate the theory to fellow participants. Some participants find the long list of theories in Box 3 confusing and time consuming to read in a single workshop, and facilitators may choose to select only two or three on the list. The idea is not to state these are the only theories with utility in IPCEP, but to develop participants' skills in selecting theories and applying these to different levels of the narrative. Facilitators emphasize that theory selection has some subjectivity, as the theory is often chosen based on the theorist's own history and familiarity, and this means that the story will be told differently dependent on theory chosen.

Box 3. Summary of Some of the Theories Applied in Workshops

Theories from sociology that explain how people behave in groups		
A focus on power relationships between groups and identity with the social group are relevant here.		
Theory	Brief Explanation	Reference
Group membership: Social Identity Theory	The theory states that we take our identity from our membership of social groups (e.g., your school class, your football club, and, in health care, your profession). In being a member of a social group we prefer to have a positive rather than a negative identity for this group. We, therefore, value and perceive the group to which we belong highly; this group is referred to as our in-group. We perceive other groups to which we do not belong less favorably, and these are referred to as our out-group. In-group bias can affect how we chose to allocate resources, in that we normally always favor our in-group.	Tajfel (1981) Tajfel and Turner (1986) Turner (1999)
Rewards of group membership: Social Capital	In socology there are many theories that look at social networks of groups. Social capital theory looks at the value of human relationships in groups. Social capital is the accumulative advantage gained from being part of a social network. It is used to understand the benefits (sometimes unequally distributed) gained by members of the group. It focuses on the value of building sustainable relationships (bonding and bridging), and how to achieve this. Social capital helps us think about norms and rules, network characteristics, internal and external resources, and trust necessary to build beneficial relationships.	Bourdieu (1997)

Theory	Brief Explanation	Reference
Power and hierarchy Expectation States Theory	Group members may predict that one particular individual in a group is more valuable than another. They defer to this individual as a result of this prediction, giving her or him more opportunities to participate. These implicit, often unconscious, anticipations of the relative quality of individual member's future performance are referred to as performance expectation and shape behavior in a self-fulfilling fashion.	Correll and Ridgeway (2003) Ridgeway (2001, 2006)

Note: For further information see Kitto et al.'s (2011) work titled *Sociology of Interprofessional Health Care and Practice*

Theories from psychology that explain individual behavior in groups
Many of these theories relate to how we form our attitudes and how our personality impacts on our behavior in groups. One branch of psychology is social psychology, bringing together research on key aspects of the individual linked to groups.

Theory	Brief Explanation	Reference
Attitude Change Contact Hypothesis	In work centered on considering why people feel hostile to one another and cannot like one another or agree, Allport (1954) proposed that when people with differences are brought together, in contact with one another, these negative perceptions are eroded. Often used as a reason for IPE, Hewstone and Brown (1986) have considered the requirements in addition to simple contact that might enable different professional groups to perceive each other favorably. Allport (1954) looked at the origins of intergroup prejudice and produced a series of influential policy recommendations. He proposed that the best way to reduce hostility between groups was to bring them together (as is proposed in IPE). However, he argued that this contact alone was not enough for positive attitude change. He, therefore, qualified his hypothesis with a number of conditions that he believed were important to the reduction of negative intergroup attitudes and stereotypes. These conditions included that each group in the contact situation should have equal status, experience a cooperative atmosphere, be working on common goals, have the support of the authorities (institutional support), be made aware of group similarities and differences, have positive expectations, and that the members of the conflicting groups perceive each other as typical members of their group.	Allport (1954) Hean and Dickinson (2005) Hewstone and Brown (1986)
Personality Myers-Briggs Inventory	The Myers-Briggs indicators measure differences between people in the way they prefer to focus their attention and energy; the way they prefer to take in information; the way they prefer to make decisions; and how they orientate themselves to the outside world. According to the theory, everyone has a natural preference for one of the opposites on each domain on each of the four dimensions (extraversion vs. introversion, sensing vs. intuition, thinking vs. feeling, and judging vs. perceiving). The theory explores our strengths and blind spots.	Briggs Myers and Myers (1995)

Note: See Bandura (1988) for further information on self-efficacy and self-belief and Festinger (1957) on cognitive dissonance theory and attitude change.

Learning theories which explain how learning takes place in groups
Learning theories focus on how the individual makes meaning or how meaning is made through social interactions; as such, these theories draw upon social and psychological theories.

Theory	Brief Explanation	Reference
Constructivist theories Experiential learning	Kolb (1984) views learning as a continuous process grounded in experience. The learner completes a cycle of learning in which experience is unpacked through reflection, analysis, and the creation of new understandings. Each step in the cycle is important in building new cognitive understandings. This learning maps to all learning styles and can be socially mediated.	Kolb (1984)
Social Constructivists Zone of Proximal Development	For these theorists, learning is not just about building new understandings; it is about how meaning is constructed through social engagement. New meaning emerges through collaborative learning. Vygotsky (1978) talks about a zone of proximal development in which learning is enabled because individuals learn with others, and this takes people beyond and into a new realm of learning.	Vygotsky (1978)

Note: See Mezirow (1997) for further information on transformative learning. Hean, Craddock, and O'Halloran's (2009) article "Learning Theories and Interprofessional Education: A User's Guide" is also recommended reading.

Organizational theories that explain the way people work together in health care
The systems where people work maybe healthcare organizations or educational institutions

Theory	Brief Explanation	Reference
Activity Theory	With its roots in social science, this theory considers a framework for considering activities that take place in complex systems. In any work system there are goals, modes of working such as divisions of labor, rules, aims, and intended outcomes. Consider when different these systems collide or come together (e.g., a nursing school coming together with a medical school to agree on IPE curriculum). There will no doubt be unresolved priorities and contradictions that emerge as members of these systems try to work together; this theory helps to unpack issues of non-alignment.	Engeström (2001)
Complex Adaptive Systems	The main aspects of a complex adaptive system consider how many elements interact with each other. Behavior in these system are often non linear and cannot be predicted.	Cilliers (1998)

Outcome frameworks
Competency frameworks are not strictly speaking a theory. However, they are a structured organized way of structuring our thought processes and providing a rationale for action.

Theory	Brief Explanation	Reference
Collaborative competencies frameworks	Competence — what individuals know or are able to do in terms of knowledge, skills, and attitude.

Capability — the extent to which individuals can adapt to change, generate new knowledge, and continue to improve their performance (Fraser and Greenhalgh 2001, p. 799):
- Role clarification/roles/responsibilities for collaborative practice
- Team functioning/interprofessional teamwork and team-based care
- Person/family/community-centered care | Canadian Interprofessional Health Collaborative (2010)

Fraser and Greenhalgh (2001)

Interprofessional Education Collaborative Expert Panel (2011) |

Theory	Brief Explanation	Reference
	• Collaborative leadership • Interprofessional communication • Interprofessional conflict resolution • Values/ethics for interprofessional practice	Walsh, Gordon, Marshall, Wilson and Hunt (2005) Wilhelmsson et al. (2012)

Note: See also Kirkpatrick's (as cited in Freeth et al. 2002) framework of educational outcomes.

Lay theories		
Your common sense way of understanding the world around you.		
Theory	Brief Explanation	Reference
Lay theory	The use of theory is not simply an academic exercise. As humans, we constantly formulate theories that later underpin our actions, even at the simplest of levels. To cross a road in our local community, for example, we put together a range of propositions: a car may approach from the right; it is likely that a car may also come from the left. If one looks left and right, the approach of car will be observed early enough to take avoiding action. We test out these hypotheses each time we cross the road and find that in most cases they prove true. The look-left-look-right theory then allow us to transfer our experiences of local roads to new contexts (e.g., a road in the busy city center).	Hean, Craddock et al. (2012)

Co-Creation of Innovative Solutions to Practice Problems Using Theory As a Tool

In small groups, participants agree as a group on one story to explore further; the story chosen generally has most relevance to them. They read the narrative in greater depth to determine whether they can identify the structure or different levels within the story (i.e., at the individual, group, organization, or society level). Practitioners and theorists then work together to reinterpret practitioner narratives through the chosen theoretical lens applied at any one of these levels. Facilitators highlight the relationship between the structure of narrative and the theory. Thus, narratives are presented as multilayered (see Box 4) and that theory can be applied to any one of these different levels to find different meanings of a single experience or story (see Box 2).

The group reviews the theory knowledge presented and then selects a relevant theory for further analysis. They can use either their own theory or a lay theory if preferred. The exercise is about theoretical skill rather than knowledge of any one theory per se. Thus, choosing a relevant theory and producing an innovative solution to the addressed practice problem in the narrative requires more than just common understanding of each other's knowledge base. It requires reaching a compromise between the political interests of both parties (i.e., theorist and practitioner, Carlile 2004). The story of the dominant participant taking precedence is one example, and the perceived status of theoretical or practice knowledge over the other is another.

Participants apply a template as they reinterpret the story using their chosen theoretical lens. To assist participants, an example of the application of a theory to the interpretations of a given narrative is provided. Participants then turn to their guided exercise using a series of trigger questions in the provided template to find new meanings to their narrative. The template guides them in considering the focus brought to the story by the theory chosen, how they have seen their story differently, and what new meaning this exercise brought to their understanding.

Box 4. Illustration given at workshop representing multilevel of narrative and multi levels at which theory can be applied

---

Narrative

The elated Girl Scout went home: her was mother proud of her for having sold all of her boxes of cookies: Those inescapable icons of capitalism, its methods and assumptions, hardwiring our children to value the power of selling in almost their every activity; the methods and assumptions are championed by some and resisted by others.

Theory can be applied at different levels
Cognition: Girl Scout's emotional state
Social development: Mother and child relationship
Society: Capitalism

Adapted from Landon, as cited in Baldwin 2013.

They are then asked to produce two questions, hypotheses, or statements that represent their new meaning of the story. A second theory may be chosen as an alternative interpretation. Participants then compare their interpretations of the narrative to observe how one or two separate theories lead to different interpretations.

Theoretical Quality and Competence

Throughout the workshop, facilitators attempt to role model dimensions of theoretical quality and make explicit the theoretical competencies being learnt. The concept of theoretical quality in the IPCEP field is discussed in greater detail elsewhere (Hean 2014, Hean et al., in review). However, in brief, theoretical quality in education, clinical, and research practice is achieved if theoretical underpinnings of our practice have been effectively articulated, operationalized, or tested within the intervention design, delivery, and assessment of outcome. The concept of theoretical quality mirrors the assessment of methodology quality used in systematic and similar literature reviews (Best Evidence Medical Education Collaboration 2012, Critical Appraisal Skills Programme 2012). Theoretical quality dimensions in IPE originate from criteria developed by Fawcett and Downs (1992, see also Fawcett 2003, 2005), and are detailed in the following sections.

Parsimony (the theory should be concisely and clearly described). For effective knowledge exchange between the theorist and practitioner, theories must be expressed in short, discrete descriptions that are clear and concise, minimizing the number of their concepts and propositions, while still capturing the basic essence of the theory. They should be described in language likely to promote shared understanding between theorist and practitioner. This is important to engage practitioners and to maintain their interest. This interest may be lost if the description of theory is overly technical and detailed.

In the workshop model, we operationalize this dimension in three ways:

- Provision of a quick overview, in which the theorist is challenged to present an oral summary of their theory of choice in a 3-minute sell. This forces the theorist to prioritize the essence of the theory as clearly and understandably as possible.
- Provision of a poster displayed on a wall of the workshop venue and in which diagrammatic representations of the theory are depicted.
- Development of crib sheets (see Box 4) that bring together brief one-paragraph summaries of each theory applied.

Positive evaluations of these resources have been provided, with some participants indicating that this was the first time a particular theory had made sense to them. However, these workshops are still evolving, and for some the written representations were still difficult to understand, especially among second-language speakers.

During the workshop presentation we explain the logic behind the 3-minute sell, poster, and crib sheets to give participants insight into the importance and skill required in making a theory clear in a minimum of times and space. This skill is something they will need to replicate when reporting and publishing their own practice in word-limited publications.

Testability (the theory must be converted into clear testable propositions or hypotheses). Practitioners must be to apply theory to their practice by developing clear research questions, propositions, and hypotheses developed from the theory. Each of these statements should have the potential to be tested empirically. In the workshops we operationalize this in two ways. First, in the poster representations, we ask facilitators to provide exemplar hypotheses or questions to demonstrate how the theory can be tested in practice. Similarly, participants are asked to produce their own hypotheses, statements, and questions (guided by a workshop template) and then show how these have been derived from a particular theory.

Empirical adequacy (research methods must be chosen that are appropriate to testing the propositions). This criterion is fulfilled if appropriate methods are used to test the propositions or questions created. For example, if social capital theory (see Box 3) is applied to a small group's story in a continuing interprofessional workshop, then the propositions developed might relate to the quality and sustainability of relationships formed between practitioners of different professions during a workshop session. To test this, a qualitative approach the facilitator explores with participants the quality and sustainability of the relationships they formed during the module. This exploration could be carried out by using focus groups or interviews that are provided a week and then a year after the workshop was completed. In their interview schedule, the following questions could be asked: "In your practitioner group, how would you describe the relationships with members from the same profession and with those from other professions? How did these relationship impact on your experience during the workshop? What did you learn from each other? What happened after the workshop? Did you see the members of your group again?"

Theoretical adequacy (the theory is supported by empirical data). The collection and analysis of research data may or may not support the chosen theory. If the theory is proven correct then it can be used to inform future practice. If not, the theory must be discarded in favor of another, or adjusted in line with research findings. To date, the latter two criteria of empirical and theoretical adequacy (the selection and application of research to test theoretical propositions) have not yet been introduced into the workshops. This is largely due to time restrictions put on workshop lengths to date. There is scope, however, to arrange a series of workshops in which participants develop hypotheses in initial workshops, reenter practice to operationalize these, and come back in subsequent sessions to discuss their findings and the empirical adequacy of their chosen theories.

Pragmatic adequacy (theories must have practical utility). Overall, when discussing theory, the theorist must make the direct application of the theory to the IPCEP context as obvious as possible.

The theorist must answer the following questions: What dimension of practice does the theory apply to, and how might the application of the theory inform the working lives of the practitioner and their decision making? For example, how can theory be used to inform the evaluation and learning outcomes of an IPE program? Facilitators stress in the workshops that use of theory cannot be an academic exercise that is, *theory for theory's sake*. It must have utility.

Summary of Workshop Model

The workshop model is designed to make participants aware of the meaning of theoretical quality and how to achieve this. As such, it provides a forum in which participants can develop theoretical competence. Competence is defined as what individuals know or are able to do in terms of knowledge, skills, and attitude (Fraser and Greenhalgh 2001, p. 799).

The workshops aim to increase participants' knowledge of a range of relevant theoretical frameworks, improve their skills to work with theorists and apply theory to their practice, and develop a positive attitude towards theory and its utility — in other words, to overcome the antipathy that is often associated with engagement in theoretical discussions.

From our experiences with the theory workshops, and in combination with the concepts of theoretical quality above, we conclude that theoretical competencies should include the following abilities:

- Understand that social meaning of an experience is transformed depending on the theory being applied.
- Understand stories have multiple levels and theories that can be applied to each of these.
- Select and apply a relevant theory to a range of experiences.
- Use theory as a reflective tool to either resolve or advance thinking on a range of IPCEP experiences.
- Articulate theory in an accessible manner tailored for the receiving audience.
- Choose and apply a range of theoretical constructs to a variety of different contexts to make alternative meaning of a single experience and hence to aid reflection and decision making in one's IPCEP.
- Understand the importance of theory to rigorous research and evidence-based practice.
- Use or develop theory to explain why IPCEP is expected to work and in what context (see Pawson and Tilley 1997).

- Articulate the characteristic of the theory chosen, its origins and history (e.g., sociology or psychology), and the historical slants this brings to the narrative.

CONCLUSION

In this chapter we have outlined the importance of theory to the field of IPCEP and have presented a workshop model through which theoretical competence in the IPCEP community can be developed. The model is, however, a work in progress. For example, clinical and policymaker knowledge has been largely missing in workshops to date. Efforts should be made to encourage practitioners and policymakers to engage in these workshops. The workshops help participants to develop new ways of looking at their practice problems and potential hypotheses. These outcomes need to be tested, and the workshop model may be developed into a series of workshops in which participants are able to also report back on their hypothesis testing in intervening practice periods.

To date, our workshops have also focused primarily on the deductive use of theory. The justification for this emphasis is the plethora of sociological and psychological theories explaining human relationships. This abundance limits the need for new approaches. However, there is space for inductive and abductive approaches as well as fostering quality grounded theory to develop theory specific to the IPCEP context.

Rigorous evaluation of the workshop model is required that goes beyond the limited surveys currently conducted at the end of each workshop iteration. These evaluations need to explore the question and transferability back into their practice settings of theoretical competencies by workshop participants, hence development of theoretical capability (Fraser and Greenhalgh 2001). It now remains for us to challenge theory enthusiasts, both within and without of the IN-2-THEORY community, to address some of the above recommendations and to replicate and develop the model in their own areas of theoretical and practice expertise.

REFERENCES

Alford, J. (2009). *Engaging public sector clients*. Basingstoke, United Kingdom: Palgrave.

Allport, G. W. (1954). *The nature of prejudice*. Reading, MA: Addison-Wesley.

Baldwin, A. (2013). *Narrative social work: Theory and application*. London, United Kingdom: Policy Press.

Bandura, A. (1988). Organizational application of social cognitive theory. *Australian Journal of Management*, 13, 275-302. http://dx.doi.org/10.1177/031289628801300210.

Barr, H., Koppel, I., Reeves, S., Hammick, M. and Freeth, D. (2005). *Promoting partnerships for health*. London, United Kingdom: Blackwell and CAIPE.

Bernstein, B. (1971). *Class, codes and control*. London, United Kingdom: Routledge.

Best Evidence Medical Education Collaboration (2012). *BEME coding sheet*. Retrieved from http://www.bemecollaboration.org/downloads/749/beme4appx1.pdf.

Bourdieu, P. (1997). The forms of Capital. In: A. H. Hasley, H. Lauder, P. Brown and A. Stuart Wells (Eds.), *Education: Culture, economy and society* (pp. 46-58). Oxford, United Kingdom: Oxford University Press.

Briggs Myers, I. and Myers, P. B. (1995). *Gifts differing: Understanding personality type.* Mountain View, CA: Davies-Black.

Canadian Institutes of Health Research (2014). http://www.cihr-irsc.gc.ca/e/193.html

Canadian Interprofessional Health Collaborative (2010). *A national interprofessional competency framework.* Retrieved from http://www.cihc.ca/files/CIHC_IPCompetencies_ Feb1210.pdf.

Carlile, P. R. (2004). Transferring, translating, and transforming: An integrative framework for managing knowledge across boundaries. *Organization Science,* 15(5), 555-568. http:// dx.doi.org/10.1287/orsc.1040.0094.

Cilliers, P. (1998). *Complexity and postmodernism.* London, United Kingdom: Routledge.

Clark, P. G. (2006). What would a theory of interprofessional education look like? Some suggestions for developing a theoretical framework for teamwork training. *Journal of Interprofessional Care,* 20, 577-589. http://dx.doi.org/10.1080/13561820600916717.

Clifton, M., Dale, C. and Bradshaw, C. (2007). *The impact and effectiveness of inter-professional education in primary care: An RCN literature review.* Retrieved from http:// www.rcn.org.uk/__data/assets/pdf_file/0004/78718/003091.pdf.

Correll, S. J. and Ridgeway, C. L. (2003). Expectation states theory. In: J. Delamater (Ed.), *Handbook of social psychology* (pp. 29-51). New York, NY: Kluwer.

Craddock, D., O'Halloran, C., McPherson, K., Hean, S. and Hammick, M. (2013). A top-down approach impedes the use of theory? Interprofessional educational leaders approaches to curriculum development and the use of learning theory. *Journal of Interprofessional Care,* 27, 65-72. http://dx.doi.org/10.3109/13561820.2012.736888.

Critical Appraisal Skills Programme (2012). *Critical Appraisal Skills Programme.* Retrieved from http://www.casp-uk.net/find-appraise-act/appraising-the-evidence.

Engeström, Y. (2001). Expansive learning at work: Toward an activity theoretical reconceptualization. *Journal of Education and Work,* 14, 133-156. http://dx.doi.org/10. 1080/13639080020028747.

Eraut, M. (2003). The many meanings of theory and practice. *Learning in Health and Social Care,* 2, 61-65. http://dx.doi.org/10.1046/j.1473-6861.2003.00045.x.

Fawcett, J. (2003). Theory and practice: A conversation with Marilyn E. Parker. *Nursing Science Quarterly,* 16, 131-136. http://dx.doi.org/10.1177/0894318403251788.

Fawcett, J. (2005). Criteria for evaluation of theory. *Nursing Science Quarterly,* 18, 131-135. http://dx.doi.org/10.1177/0894318405274823.

Fawcett, J. and Downs, F. S. (1992). *The relationship of theory and research* (2nd ed.). Philadelphia, PA: F. A. Davis.

Festinger, L. (1957). *A theory of cognitive dissonance.* Stanford, CA: Stanford University Press.

Fisher, W. R. (1987). *Human communication as narration: Toward a philosophy of reason, value, and action.* Columbia, SC: University of South Carolina Press.

Fraser, S. W. and Greenhalgh, T. (2001). Coping with complexity: Educating for capability. *BMJ,* 323, 799-803. http://dx.doi.org/10.1136/bmj.323.7316.799.

Freeth, D., Hammick, M., Koppel, I., Reeves, S. and Barr, H. (2002). *A critical review of evaluations of interprofessional education* (Occasional Paper No. 2). London, United Kingdom: LTSN-Centre for Health Sciences and Practices.

Freidson, E. (1970). *Profession of medicine: A study of sociology of applied knowledge.* New York, NY: Dodd Mead.

Hammick, M. (1998). Interprofessional education: Concept, theory and application. *Journal of Interprofessional Care*, 12(3), 323-332. http://dx.doi.org/10.3109/1356182980901412 3.

Hean, S. (2014). Developing theoretical rigour in interprofessional education. In: E. Willumsen, A. Ødegård and T. Sirnes (Eds.), *Collaboration: Theory and practice*. Oslo, Norway: Universitetsforlaget.

Hean, S., Anderson, E., Bainbridge, L., Clark, P., Craddock, D., Doucet, S., ... Oandasan, I. (2013). IN-2-THEORY – interprofessional theory, scholarship and collaboration: A community of practice. *Journal of Interprofessional Care*, 27, 88-90. http://dx.doi.org/10.3109/13561820.2012.743979.

Hean, S., Craddock, D. and Hammick, M. (2012). Theoretical insights into interprofessional education. *Medical Teacher*, 34(2), 158-160. http://dx.doi.org/10.3109/0142159X.2012.643263.

Hean, S., Craddock, D. and O'Halloran, C. (2009). Learning theories and interprofessional education: A user's guide. *Learning in Health and Social Care*, 8(4), 250-262.

Hean, S. and Dickinson, C. S. (2005). The contact hypothesis: An exploration of its further potential in interprofessional education. *Journal of Interprofessional Care*, 19, 480-491. http://dx.doi.org/10.1080/13561820500215202.

Hean, S., Hammick, M., Miers, M., Barr, H., Hind, M., Craddock, D., Borthwick, A. and O'Halloran, C. (2009). *Evolving theory in interprofessional education*. Bournemouth, United Kingdom: Bournemouth University.

Hean, S., O'Halloran, C., Craddock, D., Pitt, R., Anderson, L. and Morris, D. (2012). *A systematic review of the contribution of theory to the development and delivery of effective interprofessional curricula in medical education*. Initial Review Protocol, Proposal to Best Evidence Medical Education (BEME) Collaboration, Dundee, Scotland.

Hean, S. et al. (in review). Theoretical quality in systematic reviews. *Medical Teacher* [Submitted for publication].

Helme, M., Jones, I. and Colyer, H. (2005). *The theory-practice relationship in interprofessional education*. Retrieved from http://www.health.heacademy.ac.uk/lenses/occasionalpapers/col10007/m10235.html.

Hewstone, M. and Brown, R. J. (1986). Contact is not enough: An intergroup perspective on the "contact hypothesis." In: M. Hewstone and R. J. Brown, *Contact and conflict in intergroup encounters* (pp. 1-44). Oxford, United Kingdom: Blackwell.

IN-2-THEORY. [ca. 2010]. In: *Facebook* [Closed group]. Retrieved July 27, 2015, from https://www.facebook.com/groups/IN2THEORY.

Institute of Medicine (2015). *Measuring the impact of interprofessional education on collaborative practice and patient outcomes*. Washington, DC: Author.

Interprofessional Education Collaborative Expert Panel (2011). *Core competencies for interprofessional collaborative practice*. Retrieved from http://www.aacn.nche.edu/education-resources/ipecreport.pdf.

Jary, D. J. and Jary, J. (1995). *Collins dictionary of sociology*. Glasgow, United Kingdom: Collins.

Kolb, D. A. (1984). *Experiential learning*. Englewood Cliffs, NJ: Prentice-Hall.

Kitto, S., Chesters, J., Thistlethwaite, J. and Reeves, S. (2011). *Sociology of interprofessional health care practice: Critical reflections and concrete solutions (health care issues, costs and access)*. New York, NY: Nova Science.

Mezirow, J. (1997). Transformative learning: Theory to practice. *New Directions for Adult and Continuing Education*, 74, 5-12. http://dx.doi.org/10.1002/ace.7401.

Parsons, T. (1951). *The social system*. New York, NY: Routledge.

Pawson, R. and Tilley, N. J. (1997). *Realistic evaluation*. London, United Kingdom: Sage.

PROFRES (2014). *Forskerskolen PROFRES* [PROFRES research school]. Retrieved from https://www.uis.no/forskning-og-ph-d-studier/forskerskolen-profres/.

Reeves, S. (Ed.) (2013). [Special issue]. *Journal of Interprofessional Care*, 27(1).

Ridgeway, C. L. (2001). Gender, status and leadership. *Journal of Social Issues*, 57, 637-655. http://dx.doi.org/10.1111/0022-4537.00233.

Ridgeway, C. L. (2006). Status construction theory. In: P. J. Burke (Ed.), *Contemporary social psychological theories* (pp. 301-323). Stanford, CA: Stanford University Press.

Ridgeway, C. L. (2011). *Framed by gender*. Oxford, United Kingdom: Oxford University Press.

Tajfel, H. (1981). *Human groups and social categories*. Cambridge, United Kingdom: Cambridge University Press.

Tajfel, H. and Turner, J. C. (1986). The social identity theory of intergroup behavior. In: S. Worchel and W. G. Austin (Eds.), *The psychology of intergroup relations* (pp. 7-24). Chicago, IL: Nelson-Hall.

Turner, J. (1999). Some current issues in research on social identity and self-categorization theories. In: N. Ellemers, R. Spears and B. Doosjie (Eds.), *Social identity* (pp. 6-64). Oxford, United Kingdom: Blackwell.

Vygotsky, L. (1978). *Mind in society*. Cambridge, United Kingdom: University Press Cambridge.

Wackerhausen, S. (2009). Collaboration, professional identity and reflection across boundaries. *Journal of Interprofessional Care*, 23, 455-473. http://dx.doi.org/10.1080/13561820902921720.

Walker, D. and Nocon, H. (2007). Boundary-crossing competence: Theoretical considerations and educational design. *Mind, Culture, and Activity*, 14, 178-195. http://dx.doi.org/10.1080/10749030701316318.

Walsh, C. L., Gordon, M. F., Marshall, M., Wilson, F. and Hunt, T. (2005). Interprofessional capability: A developing framework for interprofessional education. *Nurse Education in Practice*, 5, 230-237. http://dx.doi.org/10.1016/j.nepr.2004.12.004.

Wilhelmsson, M., Pelling, S., Uhlin, L., Owe Dahlgren, L., Faresjö, T. and Forslund, K. (2012). How to think about interprofessional competence: A metacognitive model. *Journal of Interprofessional Care*, 26(2), 85-91. http://dx.doi.org/10.3109/13561820.2011.644644.

In: Interprofessional Client-Centred Collaborative Practice   ISBN: 978-1-63483-754-5
Editor: Carole Orchard   © 2015 Nova Science Publishers, Inc.

Chapter 11

EVALUATION OF CONTINUING INTERPROFESSIONAL CLIENT-CENTERED COLLABORATIVE PRACTICE PROGRAMS

Carole Orchard
Western University,
London, ON, Canada

ABSTRACT

This chapter highlights the value of developing program evaluation approaches that focus on the merit or worth of the learning in relation to the program's perceived accuracy, utility, feasibility, and propriety. A number of approaches to creating a program evaluation plan are provided. A case is made for the application of program logic models (PLMs) to continuing interprofessional education (CIPE) program evaluation. The argument is raised about the comprehensive nature in its application of an open systems approach that allows the linking back to the reason for the program.

A case study is then provided to demonstrate how a manager can apply PLM to a performance problem to build a beginning approach in designing the learning associated with needed performance change within an interprofessional team. A discussion is then provided on how the PLM approach integrates other frameworks advocated for CIPE.

INTRODUCTION

Evaluating a continuing educational program at the post-licensure level is often considered last when developing educational programs. However, it will be argued such measurement needs to be an integral component in any program development. To understand this important area, we first must define what we mean by program evaluation. Fitzpatrick, Sanders, and Worthen (2004) suggest program evaluation is "the identification, clarification, and application of defensible criteria to determine an evaluation object's value (worth or merit) in relation to criteria" (p. 5). They further identify four criteria: (a) *accuracy,* relating to the "extent to which the information obtained is an accurate reflection . . . with reality"

(Fitzpatrick et al. 2004, p. 7); (b) *utility,* relating to the "extent to which the results serve practice information needs of intended users" (p. 7); (c) *feasibility,* related to the "extent to which the evaluation is realistic, prudent, diplomatic, and frugal" (p. 7); and (d) *propriety,* "extent to which the evaluation is done legally and ethically, protecting the rights of those involved" (p. 7).

Accuracy in the context of continuing interprofessional development (CIPD) relates to ensuring the program addresses identified problematic team performance areas as viewed by the participants. As such, how well the learning activities are designed will assist in addressing and providing, where needed, additional knowledge, skill development, or exploration of underlying attitudes that may impede a change in performance. Thus, the program, in order to be accurate, must assist participants in creating plausible connections with what current practice is and how it can be viewed by them as modifiable.

Utility of the program flows from the agreement by the participants that the team's areas of performance needing enhancement, if attended to, will change practice in a realistic and beneficial way. This means they must see that there is a personal benefit to them in relation to their time and workload improvements for the program to have utility.

Feasibility of the program relates to how well the program is designed and implemented to allow for the planned outcomes to be realized given the (a) time available, (b) setting it is to be provided in, (c) facilitator who will support the learning, (d) characteristics of the participants, and (e) activities being provided to achieve the intended outcomes. When the plan can be implemented within the above it can be considered to be feasible.

Propriety relates to how the plan for feedback, assessment of learners, and evaluation of the program itself will be carried out. The processes to be adopted need to attend to the ethical issues associated with any collection of data. Participants providing the data must be assured that measures will be taken to ensure their confidentiality is maintained unless they personally choose to identify themselves. When these conditions are present the program is deemed to have propriety.

Thus, effective program evaluation planners must be cognizant of decisions reached by the program developers (who may be the same individuals) to ensure accuracy, utility, feasibility, and propriety of the program and its evaluation. They next must then consider the approach used in designing the program to identify what to evaluate. This chapter will focus on a variety of strategies that can be used to develop a CIPE program evaluation.

PROGRAM EVALUATION

The means to develop a program evaluation is founded on the decisions made in developing the program. These decisions allow for identifiers to focus on in determining the program's capacity to meet its goals or objectives. Program feasibility provides the parameters around what learning can be supported during the allotted time. Utility of the program influences the strategies that might be employed to address the means to help participants see the need for the performance change required. To gain insight, however, necessitates helping the participants understand their current practice in the chosen topic area and how it is impacting on their team's performance limitations. Then providing the means for the participants to think about new ways to address the identified limitation and be able to try out new strategies to create alternative approaches to overcome the limits that are currently interfering with high-quality care in the chosen topic, in a safe in-program role-play situation. The depth of learning chosen for the program may flow from a variety of suggested frameworks found in the literature, these being Freeth and Reeves' (2004) presage, process, and product framework; the Kirkpatrick–Barr's assessment of learning framework (Carpenter, Barnes, Dickson, and Wooff 2006, p. 148); Armitage, Connolly, and Pitt's (2008) principles for practice framework; and Greenfield, Nugus, Travaglia, and Braithwaite's (2010) interprofessional praxis audit framework (IPAF), to name a few.

In Freeth and Reeves' (2004) presage, process, and product approach, factors that influence how the program is developed, implemented, and outcomes assessed are related to the *presage* decision making. These include the context for the learning (what is the setting?) and the characteristics of the program developers (e.g., their expertise and topic of the program), the facilitators (who will deliver the program?), and of the learners (who will be the participants in the program?). While the *process* focuses on approaches being planned for the learning (what strategies are to be used to provide the knowledge, skills, and attitude shifts needed in the participants to determine success of the program) and finally the *product*. For example, the product could be client-centered interprofessional collaborative teamwork or a component within participants' teamwork (Freeth and Reeves, 2004, pp. 44–45). Hence the presage, process, and product framework provides both structural factors that lay a foundation of the program while also identifying the processes or learning activities that are provided that use the structural factors to assist in creating change within participants (Freeth and Reeves, 2004).

A further means used to guide program development is through the Kirkpatrick–Barr framework (Carpenter et al. 2006), which addresses the level of assessment desired through a learning program. Hence, it assists program developers to consider the level of outcome desired in the participants. Each level creates a higher level of learning outcome from the base of attitudinal reaction to learning all the way to change in patient care. It is comprised of four levels with two sub-levels. Level 1 focuses only on learners' reaction(s) to the learning, while Level 2a creates the need for a moderation in attitudes and/or perceptions among learners, while in Level 2b there is also an acquisition of knowledge and skills that influence these changes. Level 3 increases the learning outcome to result in changes in behaviors among the learners, thus necessitating a challenging of their assumptions and consideration of making changes in practice as a result. In the final Level 4 the focus is beyond the learner to 4a addressing changes in organizational practices and 4b in perceptible benefits to the recipients of learners' practice (Carpenter et al. 2006, p. 148). Thus, this framework will assist in determining what the focus on learning activities should be in the program — being designed. Hence, both of the above frameworks can be used in conjunction with each other. While the Freeth and Reeves' (2004) presage, process, and product framework allows for making decisions regarding a desired change based on the structural components available, the Kirkpatrick–Barr framework (Carpenter et al. 2006) allows the level of learning desired to be identified as well as the intended outcomes for the program. The principles for practice framework reported by Armitage et al. (2008) focuses on criteria that can be used as a checklist to ensure decisions are made related to the design and operationalization of the program. These include "effective coordination for strategy and implementation, recruitment and selection of [learners], development of [facilitators], [program] design, delivery and management, practice learning, assessment of learning, monitoring and review, and recruitment of [facilitators]" (Armitage et al. 2008, p. 280). Thus, these principles can be applied as a checklist during both development of and evaluation of any CIPE program.

Finally, Greenfield et al.'s (2010) IPAF is an approach to address Kirkpatrick–Barr's Level 4a. Thus, the IPAF focuses on the organization in which participants are employed and how interprofessional learning and practice is currently being demonstrated. Five components are focused on the "context, culture, conduct, attitudes, and information" (Greenfield et al. 2010, p. 437). The IPAF's interesting audit framework employs an action research approach to create the case study assessment at a unit level. The IPAF may be used as a needs assessment of interprofessional practice by teams to identify their current strengths and areas for enhancement. Thus, the IPAF allows for both a needs assessment and a means to evaluate the transfer of learning from a CIPE program into practice at a team level. The assessment of this transference will be discussed more fully in Chapter 12.

While each of the above frameworks have their strengths, they do not provide an overarching means to develop, plan, implement, and evaluate CIPE programs for their accuracy, utility, feasibility, and propriety in achievement of outcomes through a comprehensive means. A number of approaches have been proposed in the literature. All of these approaches depend on the goals for the evaluation set by the requesters of the program evaluation. Given the need to focus on the impact of change in practice from the CIPE program, one approach to assessment of practice change is through the application of a PLM. PLMs employ an open-systems approach that link the reason for the program through a series of decision points believed to be required to lead to a change in performance that is expected to resolve the beginning problem that stimulated the need for the CIPE program.

Program Logic Model Evaluation Approach

A PLM is based on program theory of change, which "defines all the building blocks required to bring about a given long-term goal" (Center for Theory of Change 2013, para. 1). Another source for PLM design is Wyatt Knowlton and Phillips' (2013) approach to PLMs, which stresses the need to focus around three key questions: "Are you doing the right work? Can you make better decisions? Are you getting superior results?" (p. 12). These questions may be applied in Greenfield et al.'s (2010) IPAF case study approach, but for the purposes of this chapter discussion we will consider the approach advocated for a group change as would be expected within interprofessional client-centered collaborative teams. According to Coffman (1999), A PLM is a depiction of a set of interrelated connections comprised of: *inputs* (what are the resources you needed for the program), *activities* (learning strategies used to achieve the program goals/objectives), *outputs* (products from the program), *short-term outcomes* (changes from the program itself), *long-term outcomes* (changes observed in practice to determine the outcomes from the learning), and *impacts* (changes in previous practice based on the program).

Logic models begin with a hoped for change that will improve the current situation. Hence, the program developers must know clearly why there is a need for the change in performance and have insight into what is the current practice. Thus, the program focuses on the gap between the current and the desired. When known, the intended change in performance achieved through the program is assumed to result in an improved outcome from what is currently present (Fitzgerald et al. 2004, p. 79). Another approach is through the application of appreciative inquiry developed by Cooperrider and Whitney (2005), in which participants are encouraged to consider what are their strengths in a given practice area and then to contemplate what their ideal practice in the area would be. The focus again for the participants is the gap between their strengths and their desire. Learning is then focusing on actions that can be taken by the team to stretch to the desired outcome. The advantage of the appreciative inquiry approach is the focus not on the team's performance problems but on existing strengths in their practice and how to build on these to gain an envisioned higher quality than just overcoming their weak area. The learning activities set out for either approach will vary.

Some may argue other factors outside of the team's practice control may influence their current performance. These may arise from organizational policies, procedures, or controls that are beyond the program being planned and may influence the level of change that can be achieved. Therefore, it is prudent for any program evaluators to state such possibilities as a limitation to practice outcomes. That being said, the needed change providing the basis for development of the educational program and identified change (outcome) remains the focus of the program evaluation.

The foundation for any logic model is the identification of needs or problems with the current practice situation. In the past, potential participants were always invited to complete a needs assessment for their own learning. The problem with this approach is the ability for potential participants to determine whether or not they have a clear understanding of what the ideal (change) in their practice could be. Hence, one's ability to identify needs is restricted by his or her own experiential knowledge. If, for example, some of the team members are new to practicing within interprofessional teams and are unfamiliar with the interprofessional collaboration competencies, they may be unable to identify, in a needs assessment, what learning they need to be able to practice within the team.

Newer approaches to collecting performance needs use literature reviews or assessment of an aspect of practice by having potential participants to complete instruments (questionnaires) that are based on theoretical concepts associated with the area for the program. Identification of needs arise from their relevant conceptual gaps in their knowledge, skills, or attitudes based on their ratings of items associated with each concept. The ratings have a greater likelihood of helping provide a mean of needs for the total team and how they view their current ability to practice in the team as compared to competence in the items.

Generally, in CIPE, the request for a program is often made by a manager or other administrator.

Thus, the perception of the gap between actual and desired practice may not be fully shared by all the potential participants. This may set a reticence of staff members to attend the CIPE session. Using the above survey approach allows the results to be shared with the participants and often creates credibility of the results with the participants. This may allow for a greater buy-in by the participants when the results are shared with them at the beginning of the program. The program is then structured to address the weakest areas identified.

This credibility arises from the fact that the data came from them. Examples of some instruments that can be used for the above purposes are provided in Chapter 12.

Survey data obtained from questionnaires can then be used to formulate learning goals that may more effectively address needs for changes than the traditional self-reported needs assessments. Using such approaches to gather information can provide a baseline of knowledge for shaping the program. Thus, general needs assessment may lack the above level of rigor and can fall short of helping to identify needed changes in practice. A case study will be provided to assist in demonstrating application of a program logic model (see Figure XV) to a continuing education program.

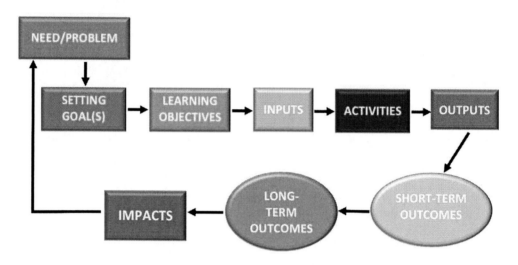

Figure XV. Program logic model components.

CASE STUDY

Charles Sawyer is an administrator of a newly established family health team in a small rural community. The team includes two family physicians, two nurse practitioners, one registered nurse, one registered dietitian, one social worker, two receptionists, and one administrator. The intent was that the team would work collaboratively to provide client-centered care. Charles arrived in his role 1 year ago and began to hear from both staff and clients that team members often did not know what other members were communicating to their clients and the same information was often being asked of the same clients.

Charles received a report about an error in care of one of their clinic clients from the regional health board representative following a complaint from a client. An error in both the client's assessment and diagnosis had occurred. This error resulted in the client being rushed by ambulance to the referral hospital Emergency Room in heart failure. Charles received the report and then brought staff involved in the incident together to discuss what might have caused this incident and what changes need to be made to ensure such an error does not occur again. It became clear that one of the physicians had seen the client and ordered puffers to resolve a breathing problem and sent the client on her way. The client returned 2 days later to report she was no better and finding her breathing more difficult. This time one of the nurse practitioners assessed her and noted swelling in her ankles and also wet rales in her chest. She sent a note to the physician about the new findings and suggested that this client needed a cardiac workup. The physician, not having worked with this nurse practitioner before, questioned her assessment and chose to continue on the previous treatment plan. Although the nurse practitioner tried to politely challenge this decision, her concerns were ignored. The receptionist also commented to the nurse practitioner that the client's husband had indicated to her that he did not feel the first treatment was 'right.'

Charles felt that the outcome of his findings from the case was a clear indication that the team was not employing collaborative practice, and staff input into discussions was not being valued or listened to by the physician. In this case, Charles was also concerned that the power being exerted over the nurse practitioner by the physician was resulting in ethical problems for the nurse practitioner. He had read in research studies that such situations could lead to turnover intent.

Charles began by starting to draw up a PLM to help him in determining how to address this teamwork problem. The outcome needed to be interprofessional client-centered collaborative practice with a particular focus on four interprofessional competencies: client- and family-centered care, interprofessional communications, team functioning, and interprofessional conflict resolution. He contacted the IPE office in the nearby university to seek assistance. Charles and the faculty member both agreed to consider asking the staff to complete two instruments: (a) the Interprofessional Socialization and Valuing Scale (King, Shaw, Orchard, and Miller 2010) that measures their socialization towards working interprofessionally and (b) the Assessment of Interprofessional Team Collaboration Scale (Orchard, King, Khalili, and Bezzina 2013) that measures the team's client-centered collaborative practice. Charles approached the staff to ask if they would be willing to complete these instruments. He was surprised that all staff agreed. They commented that they wanted to ensure another error in care did not occur. The outcome of this assessment identified their attitudes towards working with each other were interfering with their socialization towards wanting to work together, and their partnership with their clients and each other as well as cooperation amongst team members were also weak areas. After further consultation, the IPE expert at the university suggested that Charles and his staff pick only one area to focus on first. The staff felt that their cooperation with each other was the most important area to work on. Charles then asked staff members if they would like to help in developing the program. Two members indicated their willingness (a nurse practitioner and a family physician).

The first step in developing the PLM was to identify the change that they wanted to see in their team practice. The planning group felt they wanted to be more client and family focused, and to be valued by all team members for the knowledge, skills, and expertise they bring into care planning within the collaborative team. They also wanted to explore ways to include clients and family members more in their care. This meant that two foci would be considered:

- Goal #1: Collaborative teamwork with each other.
- Goal #2: How to include clients and family members in their care.

In the next step they needed to consider what learning objectives would be needed to achieve each goal. The learning outcomes for Goal #1 resulted in identification of seven learning objectives:

1. To gain an understanding of what constitutes interprofessional cooperative team practices.
2. To discuss how to apply cooperation to their teamwork.
3. To identify what they already do to support cooperative team practices.

4. To identify what they would like to see demonstrated in the team to support cooperative team practices.
5. To assess the gap between current cooperation in the team and what would be the ideal.
6. To determine what action they will take to overcome the gap.
7. To choose how they will assess when the ideal cooperative teamwork is demonstrated.

The planning group began with the first learning objective and considered what *inputs* (resources) they would need to be able to achieve this objective. Resources they identified included (a) literature about cooperation in team working that would identify the knowledge, skills, and attitudes needed for the team to be able to achieve the goal; (b) the clinic staff to participate in a team-building program; (c) a facilitator with expertise in teamwork cooperation to support the learning; (d) time release from providing care to deliver the program so all staff could participate; (e) a place to hold the learning sessions; (f) flip charts and markers; (g) a projector and laptop computer; (h) learning materials; and (i) data related to team cooperation from the baseline survey.

Next the planning group sought a meeting with the interprofessional expert from the university IPE office to assist in helping them to consider what *learning activities* would help to achieve their objective. The IPE expert explored with them three key areas: (a) setting principles for working with each other; (b) understanding each other's roles, knowledge, skills, and expertise; and (c) creating guidelines for communicating with each other and dealing with disagreements. Each of these areas was considered as a learning activity in the PLM. Their university colleague guided the planning group in how to develop their learning activity by exploring the first key area — setting principles for working with each other. She shared one potential strategy they could use. This strategy applies a modified nominal group process in which each staff member is asked to write down on a post-it note (using one note per idea) how they want to be treated by each other, then all staff share their ideas and post these on a flip chart. The group is encouraged to identify and eliminate duplications and have staff members rate the most important remaining items to them by using five votes each. The facilitator then adds up the votes and the top five ideas are translated into statements that reflect what the team's principles are for working with each other. The members are then encouraged to use these principles to hold each other accountable as to how they behave with each other.

Charles realized that these steps also help to identify the *outputs* for this objective, that is the development of a set of principles for working with each other and also looking at a way to track when staff have used reminders with each other about the principles. This then led the planning group considering what should be the *short-term outcomes* for this objective. Planning group members suggested development of a short checklist for staff to complete to record each time they used the principles with each other, and further they could create a simple questionnaire to rate on a 5-point ratings scale (from 1 = not at all to 5 = all the time) their perceptions of how they feel respected, listened to, and valued for their expertise. This assessment would be carried out once a year on an ongoing basis, and the results would be reported back to all staff. They then considered how to determine what the *long-term outcomes* should be. They finally came up with the idea that if staff really cooperated with each other in the team, then no one would want to leave the team, so turnover would be one indicator. They had also heard that absenteeism should decrease and, therefore, could be assessed by Charles and reported back to the team annually as well. The planning group also noted that, since they are a relatively new team, it will be difficult to do a comparison from before their current practices in these areas, but the current figures would be used as the standard against which to assess the future rates.

Finally the *impact* of team changes in cooperating with each other could be assessed by asking their clients and family members about how well the staff members work with each other, and in supporting their care. Thus, Charles and the planning group had worked through one of activities for one of the learning objectives within one of the goals set. Their complete PLM would take more time to develop. He also knew that this was just the start of the process for transforming his clinic group into a client-centered and collaborative team.

DISCUSSION

Within the above case study the inputs equate to the presage in the Freeth and Reeves' (2004) framework, while the activities relate to Levels 2a, 2b, 3, and 4b from Kirkpatrick-Barr's assessment learning framework (Carpenter et al. 2006, p. 148).

This example also focused on several of the principles for practice advocated by Armitage et al. (2008). The location of the case also allows the impact to assist in determining an aspect of interprofessional practice associated with Greenfield et al.'s (2010) IPAF.

Hence the above discussion and example of the application of a PLM provides a means for evaluating a continuing interprofessional education program. Furthermore, the PLM for evaluating the program also meets the four criteria set out by Fitzpatrick et al. (2004): (a) *accuracy*, identifying a real problem in the practice environment provides an accurate focus for the program; (b) the program will have *utility* since the learning provided will address changes in practice needed to improve client care; (c) the program's *feasibility* will be achieved by assessing the impact of the team performance change using practical and available evidence identified by the planning group and based on team's data results; and (d) the evaluation will have *propriety,* since collection of evidence about the change is designed to solicit information without coercion from those involved either in making the change or as recipients of the change.

CONCLUSION

CIPE without attention to well-designed program evaluation limits the ability to ensure the design of the program is based on available resources, with learning activities flowing from participants' identified weaknesses in performance, and assessed against short-term evaluation of goal achievement. The transfer of learning into team practice is then evaluated as a long-term outcome that is compared with change in team performance from the reason for the CIPE program. In the next chapter the focus will shift to the assessment of the learning within each individual.

REFERENCES

Armitage, H., Connolly, J., and Pitt, R. (2008). Developing sustainable models of interprofessional learning in practice – the TUILIP project. *Nurse Education in Practice 8*, 276–282. http://dx.doi.org/10.1016/j.nepr.2007.10.004

Carpenter, J., Barnes, D., Dickson, C., and Wooff, D. (2006). Outcomes of interprofessional education for Community Mental Health Services in England: The longitudinal evaluation of a postgraduate programme. *Journal of Interprofessional Care, 20*, 145 – 161. http://dx.doi.org/10.1080/13561820600655653

Center for Theory of Change. (2013). *What is theory of Learning from logic models: An example of a family/school partnership program.* Harvard Family Research Project. http://hugs1.harvard.edu/~hfrp.

Cooperrider, D. L., and Whitney, D. (2005). *Appreciative inquiry a positive revolution in change.* San Francisco, CA: Berrett-Koehler.

Fitzpatrick, J. L., Sanders, J. R., and Worthen, B. R. (2004). *Program evaluation: Alternative approaches and practice guidelines* (3rd ed.). Boston, MA: Pearson Education.

Freeth, D., and Reeves, S. (2004). Learning to work together: Using the presage, process, product (3P) model to highlight decisions and possibilities. *Journal of Interprofessional Care, 18*, 43–56. http://dx.doi.org/10.1080/13561820310001608221

Greenfield, D., Nugus, P., Travaglia, J. and Braithwaite, J. (2010). Auditing an organization's interprofessional learning and interprofessional practice: The interprofessional praxis audit framework (IPAF). *Journal of Interprofessional Care, 24*(4), 436–449. DOI: 10.3109/13561820903163801

King, G., Shaw, L, and Orchard, C.A., and Miller, S. (2010). The interprofessional socialization and valuing scale: A tool for evaluating the shift toward collaborative care approaches in health care settings. *Work: Journal of Prevention, Assessment and Rehabilitation.*

Orchard. C., King, G., Khalili, and Bezzina, M.B. (2012). Assessment of Interprofessional Collaborative Practice (AITCS): Development and testing of the instrument. *Journal of Continuing Education in the Health Professions, 32*(1), 58-67. DOI: 10.1002/chp.21123.

Wyatt, Knowlton, L., and Phillips, C. C. (2013). *The logic model guidebook: Better strategies for great results.* Thousand Oaks, CA: Sage.

Chapter 12

ASSESSMENT OF LEARNING WITHIN INTERPROFESSIONAL CLIENT-CENTERED COLLABORATIVE PRACTICE – CHALLENGES AND SOLUTIONS

Carole Orchard

Western University, London, ON, Canada

ABSTRACT

The focus in this chapter is on the assessment of learning associated with continuing interprofessional education (CIPE) programs. It presents a case for using a formative approach to learning that is then assessed beyond just the CIPE program. How a participant converts learning gained and how it can be shared with fellow members in an interprofessional team are discussed. Factors that influence and impede knowledge uptake are presented. The chapter then shifts to discussion of assessment of team performance addressing team dynamics, knowledge contributions of members, and the organizational environment within which the team practices. Finally, the author provides examples of measurement instruments that can be used for an organization to determine the level of interprofessional client-centered collaboration in teams that is present across a variety of service areas.

Keywords: Assessment, formative learning, life-long learning, shared knowledge, shared learning, learning transfer

INTRODUCTION

We often use the terms evaluation and assessment to mean the same processes when considering measurement of the learning participants gain from a CIPE program. However, assessing learning relates to the formative or ongoing development of learning as one gains more knowledge, skills, and insights. Assessment of learning is used for certification of learning (summative) and to help with one's learning at a key point in time (formative). For the purposes of this chapter we are focusing on the latter or formative learning. The relevancy of this focus relates to the ongoing (life-long) learning in practice that must occur at the post-licensure level to assist practitioners to be, as Bleakley (2006) discusses, "fit for practice." Bleakley challenges a focus on only the learning that occurs within the CIPE program by presenting the importance of the "sociocultural models of learning, where the learner is viewed as subject of social and historical discourse, and cognition is described as distribution across people and artefacts making up a community of practice, rather than situated in persons" (p. 151). He further stresses the importance of the information flow between members in a team (Bleakley 2006). It appears that knowing within oneself is insufficient until it is shared with others through interactions, allowing for a participation in knowledge expansion or conversely contraction, which is there stored not as a solitary knowing but as a team's "rememberings"; the learning then becomes a "jointly realized activity" (Bleakley 2006, pp. 152–153). If we support the above, then restricting assessment of learning to only an individual participant and to only the outcome of the learning from the CIPE program seems limited.

Participation in a CIPE program needs to be considered as the stimulus for a formative process of learning that creates opportunity for sharing of what is learned, and assessing its applicability into interprofessional team practice through the learning transfer to make judgments about how it can benefit team practice. Boud (2000) suggests formative learning today needs to be structured to allow the learner to determine if the 'standard' set out by the program is being met. The Interprofessional Collaboration Competencies shared by Orchard and Bainbridge (in Chapter 2) provide one form of standard that can be used. These standards may be transformed as CIPE program learning objectives. Further, it is important to determine whether the learning has merit to one's practice. If the learning is of value to the CIPE program participants, then participants' formative assessment of the learning as an outcome from the CIPE program is dependent on individuals sharing their learning with team members (Boud 2000). This sharing with team members relates to Bainbridge and Reghr's (Chapter 4) learning network, and, as Bender et al. (Chapter 9) suggest, the team then becoming a community of inquiry will enable application of the learning into their shared experimentation. Trialing the learning in practice is then followed by their team assessment of its effectiveness and determination for continuance, for adjustment, or for deletion of the trial change depending on shared feedback obtained. Hence, in this chapter, a cycle is provided related to assessment of learning beginning with a CIPE program, then moving into the transfer process of the learning gained by the learner into knowledge that can be shared, and its uptake by the team, followed by a commitment to trial the new knowledge and determine if the quality of their teamwork and its impact on their clients care improves (or does not improve).

Learning Assessment

Assessment of the learning gained from a continuing interprofessional education program is generally gained through feedback from participants on their learning experience using a feedback — or what is often termed 'evaluation' — form. However, the connection between the learning gained from the program and how it was transferred into practice and more importantly whether any change was sustained as an outcome is often not carried out. Hence a key focus is determining if the learning gained at the end of an educational session translates and is then applied to their practice and finally results in a positive health outcome for clients.

Assessment of learning focuses on the learning achieved by those who participated in the program. Hence, this assessment focuses on the individual or group of individuals working collaborative together. When assessment is considered at the continuing education level it reflects three levels of assessment. The first level, and the most commonly focused on, is the professional level, and it relates directly to both the entry-to practice competencies professionals are expected to have as they set out into practice, and their ongoing practice monitored through enacting standards of practice and codes of ethics set out within each profession. The second level relates to individual professionals as members of an interprofessional team and how they participate within the team. Criteria for this level can be considered as the interprofessional competencies ascribed through the 2010 Canadian Interprofessional Health Collaborative (CIHC) *National Interprofessional Competency Framework* (patient/client/family/community-centered care, interprofessional communication, role clarification, team functioning, interprofessional collaborative leadership, and interprofessional conflict resolution) or the Interprofessional Education Collaborative (2011) *Core Competencies for Interprofessional Collaborative Practice* (values/ethics for interprofessional practice, roles/responsibilities, interprofessional communication, and teams and teamwork).

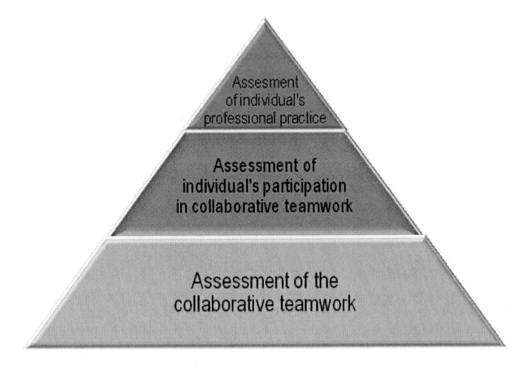

Figure XVI. Interprofessional levels of assessment for teamwork.

Hence, at this level, professionals are enacting both their professional and interprofessional competence to practice within a team. At the third level the focus is on the team and its collaborative functioning. Again the two sets of competencies identified for the second level can be applied, but addressing how the total collaborative group works together. Some promising work is being carried out by the CIHC International Interprofessional Competency Work Group through their Interprofessional Collaborative Team Judgment Process Assessment Tool framework (Orchard, Anderson, Ford, and Moran, 2015). This framework is comprised of five sequential phases (getting ready, working together to assess, diagnose and plan care, delivery care, and reviewing care) and one integrated phase (reflecting on teamwork throughout the process). Within each of these phases the processes that are expected to occur relate to each of the CIHC competencies being identified (Orchard 2015). The focus of discussion on assessment in the remainder of this chapter will focus on both Levels 2 and 3 (see Figure xiv).

Measurement of the Individual Member, or of the Team?

Measurement is generally considered to be about performance by individuals within a job role. However, it is presented in this chapter as occurring formatively within three dimensions of learning: (a) the learning gained from a CIPE program, (b) learning from a CIPE program and its transfer into individual practice, and (c) the impact of that transferred learning into the interprofessional client-centered collaborative team practice.

Learning As an Outcome of Continuing Interprofessional Education Training

This is the traditional level that most CE facilitators focus on and is associated with participants' session satisfaction with less emphasis on what they specifically learned in favor of global open-ended questions about its value to their learning. It is proposed here that two simple additions can enhance CIPE evaluations. Firstly, all CIPE programs have a set of objectives. These objectives are used by the session developers to guide what learning is facilitated.

Therefore, these objectives should provide insight into what was actually learned. If the objectives are taken and transformed into learning statements by the program assessors, a more in-depth understanding of what was learned can be obtained. When these statements then have a 5-point rating scale attached to each, the learning outcomes can be numerically assessed and analyzed using descriptive statistics. An example is shown below.

The values participants select for each item can then be added together and a construct of the perceived learning effectiveness of the session can be achieved as a percentage out of a possible total (in our example the total would be out of 10 items with a maximum rating of 5, for a sum of 50). If the total gained from all the participants was 45/50 then the learning effectiveness score would be 90%. Gaining information about the learning perceived to be gained from the participants is far more valuable to the CIPE facilitator than the traditional approach of only a global learning assessment of how satisfied they are with the arrangements and the program itself.

Comparison of CIPE Session Learning Objectives and their Rating as an Outcome from the Session

LEARNING OBJECTIVE	LEARNING OUTCOME*
To explore their own understanding of the roles, knowledge, and skills of selected members of interprofessional teams they normally encounter in practice settings.	I now understand how my previous socialization into my profession may have related to some myths about other health professions. I now have a better appreciation of why it is difficult to change practice from multidisciplinary to interprofessional.
To challenge their existing assumptions about interprofessional collaborative practice, including the role of the client and family within care planning.	I now understand how my previous professional education can result in problems with communications across health professions. I now have a better understanding of the role of patients/clients and families within interprofessional collaborative teams.
To explore evidence-based practice on effective interprofessional teaching strategies in practice settings.	I have gained some ideas about strategies to assist learners to be more interprofessional and collaborative.
To develop a process for assisting students in combining both professional and interprofessional learning into their practice placement learning goals.	I now have an understanding of how I can seek out practice-based interprofessional learning opportunities for students/practitioners. I have gained some ideas about actions that can be used to support interprofessional learning strategies.
To explore the means to assess interprofessional learning, including socialization changes, collaborative working relationships, client-centered care, collaborative leadership, shared decision making, and addressing conflicts in practice.	I now have an understanding of what competencies comprise interprofessional collaborative practice. I have gained an understanding of how the interprofessional competency descriptors can be used to assess interprofessional practice learning.
To explore evidence to determine students' abilities to demonstrate Interprofessional collaboration competencies at the appropriate level of their program.	I have gained an understanding of how to identify evidence that can be used to support evaluation of learners' collaborative practice.

Note. *Each statement is rated by participants using the following scale: 1 = strong disagree, 2 = disagree; 3 = neither agree nor disagree; 4 = agree; 5 = strongly agree.

The second augmentation can be in the form of additional open-ended statements or questions than in traditional feedback forms that ask about what they liked or did not about the program. In our interprofessional office we use the following standard questions on all our program evaluations:

- What surprised you the most from this learning event?
- What is the most significant thing, to you, that you will take away from this learning event?
- Overall, how would you rate this learning event? (This last question is rated by participants using a scale from 1 = of limited value to 5 = very valuable.)

Surprisingly, we receive a large number of comments to these questions that are very valuable in understanding how our participants perceived the learning event.

At this juncture participants' acquisition of new knowledge is retained within themselves. While valuable to one's own practice in a health care teamwork environment, this can limit how one's own ideas for changes in practice can be enacted.

As Bleakley (2006) discussed, the knowledge gained must be shared within the team for transfer of the learning to be fully operationalized into practice.

Transfer of Learning into Practice

In CIPE it is as important to know how the participants in a learning session transfer the learning from a CIPE session into their practice as from the program itself. The transition of learning from a CIPE session then is related to how the learner uses knowledge gained and transfers this knowledge to others in the team. As Janhonen and Johanson (2011) noted, knowledge can be *explicit* (formulated and presented in work or pictorial renderings); *implicit* (associated with the senses and tactile feelings, values, etc.); or *converted* (shared and new knowledge is created through a synthesis of explicit and tacit knowledge). The capacity of a learner to share gained knowledge is dependent on her or his capacity to synthesize both the explicit and tacit knowledge acquired. Thus, moving the learning into an understandable form through a knowledge-conversion process is needed before team members can consider integrating the new information or process. Janhonen and Johanson (2011) suggest conversion of knowledge occurs through four processes: socialization, externalization, internalization, and combined externalization-internalization (p. 218; see below).

Comparison of Knowledge Conversion into Use Within Teams

KNOWLEDGE CONVERSION PROCESSES	TRANSFER OF KNOWLEDGE	TEAM USE
SOCIALIZATION	TACIT → TACIT	Group tacit knowledge needed for task completion and group performance
EXTERNALIZATION	TACIT → EXPLICIT	Movement of ideas and images into words/concepts leading to reflection and sharing
INTERNALIZATION	EXPLICIT → TACIT	Making meaning out of ideas and images
COMBINATION-INTERNAL/ EXTERNALIZATION	TRANSFER OF CONTENT AND STRUCTURES → USABLE FORMS	Systemization of knowledge into teamwork

Note. Adapted from "Role of Knowledge Conversion and Social Networks in Team Performance" by M. Janhonen and J.-E. Johanson, 2011, *International Journal of Information Management, 31*, p. 218.

The success of an individual team member's sharing of new knowledge is dependent upon how well the knowledge is converted into the mental models that the team members share. Mental models "are organized knowledge structures that allow individuals to interact with their environment" (Mathieu, Heffner, Goodwin, Salas, and Cannon-Bowers 2000, p. 274).

The challenge for the individual in knowledge sharing is in her or his capacity to translate the knowledge gained through a profession-specific set of terms and approaches into interprofessional shared information (Pearson and Pandya 2006). The effectiveness of this sharing of information and the subsequent developing of shared mental models within the team can be assessed within the integration, synthesizing, and sharing of information and coordination of the team members' learning and how it leads to their cooperation around care task demands (Salas, Cooke, and Rosen 2008). The above elements then are critical to tracking the transfer of learning from a CIPE session into team practice and subsequent performance.

As Lamb, Wong, Vincent, Green, and Sevdalis (2011) noted, the uptake of the learning by the team can be viewed through how the team uses information they obtain (interprofessional communication), how team leadership (interprofessional collaborative leadership) is provided, and the application of team-shared decision-making processes (team functioning). Team decision-making processes can be assessed further for both the "level of involvement of different professional groups [and their] ability to reach and implement a decision" (Lamb et al. 2011, p. 3). Lavé's (2009) social learning theory may assist in considering how to assess for the uptake of the new learning in the team. Lavé considers how practitioners who come together bring with them "knowledge of different things" (p. 206), "communicate from a base of different interests" (p. 206), and bring "experiences from different social locations" (p. 206) into the same situation. In so doing, coming to a shared understanding will likely create conflicting viewpoints (interprofessional conflict resolution). The effectiveness of their collaborative teamwork then must reflect their ability to come to a shared viewpoint about the care needs of their clients (interprofessional collaborative leadership). Hence, it is the social world (practice context) and the experiences team members gain through their respective worlds that provides the enriched capacity of a collaborative team to arrive at approaches to addressing client goals. At the same time, when another individual provides her or his viewpoint into potential changes to how the team functions, unless there is an agreed-upon process for dealing with divergent viewpoints across members, the ability of the learner to influence new knowledge uptake may be at odds with team norms.

Assessing for the effectiveness of knowledge transfer may be considered by asking team members to rate their effectiveness and consider the application of their innovation to their practice Field and West's (1995) Team Effectiveness subscale on innovation may serve as a means to help in assessing this process as well as asking team members about what the new knowledge and its application to their practice means to team care delivery. Such a question may allow for the surfacing of mental models and their consistency across the team.

Further factors to consider related to transfer of learning in the team relates to members' capacity to attend to what is being discussed by the CIPE program participant, which is also influenced by 'noise' in the environment. This noise may arise from distractions occurring outside of the team, such as pressing workload that still needs to be carried out, or from a concerning problem in their personal lives that cause changes in their ability to attend to the team discussions.

Hence, perception of what is being said, often considered as effective listening, is normally challenged by noise. Lavé (2009) suggests this is normal in any environment, and strategies are needed to both attend to what the individual is sharing while providing space for other members' sharing their viewpoints about the information, which will allow for an agreement on whether or not to uptake the information and transform this knowledge into their team practice.

There is also the need to verify what team decisions are reached as an outcome of this discussion.

The process and outcome of this sharing of learning by the CIPE participant is further influenced by the culture set within and by the team, which creates a set of norms for its practice. Norms are standards that are created and shared by team members to set a tone for teamwork. How team members perceive and then enact these norms occurs at two levels — *conscious* and *unconscious*.

Unconsciously, members synthesize what is occurring in their teamwork, and this is consciously used through members emulating and actualizing perceived team norms (Pollard, 2008, p. 4). Hence, at an unconscious level, what their colleague is sharing about her or his new learning may be discounted without realizing it by some members, while others may listen and consider the information at a conscious level. Thus, there may be a need to explore the meaning of discounted viewpoints to gain more clarity as to why some members unconsciously thwart a move to change practice that others may want to enact. Periodic focus group interviews could be carried out, in which members are asked to identify issues that occurred within the team that they personally felt challenged their own perspectives and why; this may uncover how well the transfer of knowledge was then transformed (or not transformed) into a team mental model.

Clearly, the transfer of knowledge into a team environment is a complex process influenced by a variety of factors. Many of which may be out of the control of an individual trying to influence a positive change in her or his team practice. Hence, the capacity of the individual to influence a change in the performance of the team is dependent on many factors, as well as on the individual's capacity to persuade, negotiate, and adapt the new knowledge into the team. Subsequently, it is the team's performance that is the measure of the success of knowledge transfer into practice.

Assessment of Team Performance

The transfer of learning into a team seems to be associated with how the team functions. Hence, the discussion will now shift to addressing the assessment of collaborative team effectiveness. Kvarnström (2008) suggests such assessment should focus on *team dynamics, knowledge contribution from each provider*, in concert with the *organizational environment* (p. 194).

Team dynamics. Team dynamics is a commonly stated term, but what it constitutes for purposes of team assessment is somewhat amorphous. To assist, we first need to consider what a team is. Cohen and Bailey (1997) define a team as

> a collection of individuals who are interdependent in their tasks, who share responsibility for outcomes, who see themselves and who are seen by others as an intact social entity embedded in one or more larger social systems, and who manage their relationship across organizational boundaries. (p. 241)

Thus, three criteria to assess are team *interdependencies, complementary relationships*, and how they work within professional and organizational *boundaries*.

Assessment of interdependencies can be considered in relation to how well team members communicate with each other, coordinate client care with each other, and negotiate with each other, with their clients, and their clients caregivers around the most effective care feasible. Interdependencies also relate to how relationships are complementary across the team and with the team and their clients and caregivers. Gittell, Godfrey, and Thistlethwaite's (2013) approach to relational coordination can assist in identifying what to assess, for example how well the team (a) reaches shared goals with each other and with their clients and caregivers; (b) share their knowledge with each other; (c) demonstrates mutual respect for each other and for their clients and caregivers; and (d) perceives and respects boundaries of knowledge, skills, and expertise within the group. To respect boundaries, the team requires clarity in understanding the roles, knowledge, skills, and expertise of each member (role clarification), including that of their clients and their caregivers (client/family-centered care). Thus, the above become criteria for assessing team dynamics (team functioning). Consequently, using the CIHC (2010) *Interprofessional Competency Framework* provides a means for determining how the team members enact their team dynamics in practice.

Another approach to assessment of team dynamics might be achieved by taking the five dysfunctions of teams advocated by Lencioni (2002) and changing these into positive functions; for example, (a) focus on achievement of collective team results; (b) hold one another accountable; (c) commit to shared decisions and plans of action; (d) engage together in addressing and resolving conflicts around care/treatment issues; and (e) trust one another. Furthermore, Jeffery, Maes, and Bratton-Jeffery (2005) suggest that the objectives relating to team performance should focus on the following:

- Clarify their team goals, tasks, working environment, and client care needs.
- Establish the roles and responsibilities and accountabilities to which each member agrees.
- Determine how team members share information, and compare what, how, and when members communicate with each other against their agreed-upon interprofessional guidelines.
- Ascertain how the team as a whole takes advantage in sharing team members' knowledge, skills, and expertise.
- Assess how the team functions collaboratively as a team.

Thus, there are a number of criteria that can be adopted to measure client-centered collaborative teamwork effectiveness. How well team members work together, then, is dependent on the contribution that each member brings into the collaborative teamwork.

Knowledge contribution of members. The contributions of knowledge from each team member in their various forms influence the effectiveness of collaborative teamwork and create a value-added nature to team assessment. Team members' individual contributions reflect two constructs — *feelings about communicating with each other* and *means used to communicate with each other*. Field and West (1995) suggest five principles to focus on feelings relating to communication by assessing how (a) individuals feel their contributions are leading to team success; (b) individuals feel that their roles within the team are both meaningful and intrinsically rewarding to them; (c) individuals feel that the tasks they are provided to perform in the team are interesting to them; (d) the contributions of individuals are being identified, acknowledged, and assessed within the team; and (5) individuals understand team goals and how their work will be assessed against the same. Hence, it is not only the performance of the individual within the team (competence), but also how the team members make them feel about their contributions to the team (relationships) that are equally important to team effectiveness.

Relationships are about communication and interactions with each other. Thus, the *communication means* used within interprofessional collaborations to be valued should reflect the following set actions reported from Robinson, Gorman, Slimmer, and Yudkowsky's (2010) study of nurse–physician interactions: (a) provide clarity and precision in messages that are verified by members; (b) collaboratively problem-solve through respecting, soliciting, and using each other's advice; (c) maintain a calm and supportive demeanor in shared conversations even during times of stress; (4) maintain respect for each other, which leads to team trust; and (5) demonstrate authentic understanding of the unique role each member, including clients and their caregivers, contribute (p. 211). Thus, there are some principles and concepts that can be used to determine what to assess in relation to team performance effectiveness.

When assessing team performance effectiveness, assessors must consider whether they wish to focus on the process or outcomes of team functioning. In practice, a manager may wish to consider the team's performance from a formative perspective, but may also be required by the organization to provide an outcome or summative perspective at key points in time. The formative focus of team assessment, then, is on what actions the team and its members take with their clients and the client's family members to reach agreed-upon goals. Hence, assessors are advised to review Schön's (1991) stage of "reflecting-in action" (p. 49) about practice. The evaluation of team outcomes in a summative assessment relates to Schön's "reflecting-on" (p. 277) practice. That is, did the team achieve its set shared goals for a client's care. Since both process and outcomes assessments provide complementary perspectives on team performance, Salas, Rosen, Burke, Nicholson, and Howse (2007) suggest that assessment of team performance should reflect both *process* and *outcome* determinations that are carried out over time. Thus, the value of these dual assessments is in learning both about the strength of the teamwork being provided and achieved, as well as areas where further CIPE can be provided to enhance team performance.

Using either processes (formative) or outcomes (summative) goals to determine team performance judgments is dependent on how an assessor understands both the social (team) environment being assessed and the clarity of and sharing of information occurrences between team members. How an assessor perceived the situational 'reality' of the teamwork, and how the assessment is compared against the assessor's perceived norms of practice, is subject to the perspective of the assessor (Dowding and Thompson 2003). While the idea of assessing a team's collaborative work is appealing, the reality of achieving an accurate rating may be more difficult to achieve due to variances in assessors' perspectives. Clearly, standards are needed against which assessors can compare team performance to potentially arrive at consistent ratings.

Process assessment allows for understanding the sequential method that an individual in a team, or a team as a whole, used to arrive at the decision or judgment (Salas et al. 2007). Learning about the processes teams use provides insight into both the knowledge and behaviors used by team members to accomplish team tasks, whereas outcomes provide an end result of these processes (Salas et al. 2007, p. B79). The ability of collaborative teams to enact client-centered collaborative teamwork is also influenced by the support they are provided within their organization.

Organizational environment. Although a number of authors have discussed the impediments to collaborative practice at the institutional level, less attention has been focused on what can be assessed to determine a supportive environment. At the big-picture level, Légaré et al. (2011) suggest there is both a *transition zone* between the team and the organization and the *environment* set by the organization. In the transition zone, the organizational routines determine the level support for collaborative team practice, while the organizational policies, values, rules, resources, and culture create the environment that is viewed by team members as supportive or not (Légaré et al. 2011, p. 22). San Martín-Rodríguez, Beaulieu, D'Amour, and Ferrada-Videla (2005) previously identified two broad areas — *organizational determinants* and *interactional determinants* — that influence how an organization supports collaboration (p. 143). Organizational determinants relate to the leadership and expertise shown by management responsible for the team, as well as the provision of training in collaborative client-centered practice for team members, and further provision of structural supports, such as time release and funding to support team development. At the interactional determinant level, the focus is on managers to whom teams report and how they mentor, support, incorporate new knowledge and additional resources, and encourage collaborative work of teams. In more recent work, D'Amour, Goulet, Labadie, San Martín-Rodríguez, and Pineault (2008) have identified a four-dimensional model of collaboration. Two dimensions related to the organizational level (*governance* and *formalization*) and the other two to the team level (*shared goals and vision* and *internalization*). Within the governance dimension four indicators (*centrality, leadership, support for innovation*, and *connectivity*) are proposed that may provide a means to assess the impact of the organizational environment on support for the effectiveness of a collaborative team. Centrality relates to how the institutional governance sets direction to support a culture of client-centered collaborative practice. Direction is associated with the allocation of resources for both staff training and teamwork practice. While the direction is important, administrators also need to encourage, support, and celebrate with these teams for their innovations as they work to shape their unique model of client-centered collaborative practice. The administration must also facilitate cross-departmental/service connectivity to ensure collaborative teams are able to respond quickly and comprehensively to their clients' care and treatment needs. Furthermore, the formalization dimension necessitates organizations working across institutional sectors to create the means (written and agreed-upon protocols, information sharing, and resource sharing) for teams to share responsibilities for clients' care and treatments and outcomes with others outside their respective institution. Thus, having health providers in their teams and managers of the teams rate the above governance and formalization indicators could provide a self-assessment of the organizational support for their teamwork.

The organizational support for teamwork rating along with team effectiveness ratings must be compared to accurately determine how supportive their organization is to interprofessional client-centered collaborative teams and their practice. When teams assess their organization to not be in support of teamwork, their ability to enact effective teamwork may be compromised.

Comparison of Instrument for Measurement to Interprofessional Teamwork by Focus of Measurement and Concepts Assessed

NAME OF INSTRUMENT	FOCUS OF MEASUREMENT	CONCEPTS ASSESSED	SOURCE
Attitudes Health Professionals (AHPQ)	Focus on the attitudes health professionals have about themselves and other professions.	Caring (13 items), internal consistency 40.91 Subservient (7 items), Internal consistency 40.91 Cronbach α 0.75	Lindqvist, Duncan, Shepstone, Watts, and Pearce (2005)
Attitude Toward Health Care Teams (ATHCT)	Focus on general attitudes health professionals have about teams.	Quality of Care/Process (14 items), Cronbach α 0.83 Physician Centrality (6 items) Cronbach α 0.75	Heinemann, Schmidtt, Farrell and Brallier (1999)
Interprofessional Socialization and Valuing Scale (ISVS)	Focus on individual's socialization towards working interprofessionally. Also focuses on client/family involvement in teamwork.	Comfort in working with others (6 items) Self-perceived Ability to work with others (9 items) Valuing working with others (9 items) Cronbach α 0.79 to 0.89.	King, Shaw, Orchard, and Miller (2010)
Team Climate Inventory	Focus on how team members rate their team environment.	Team participation (12-items) Cronbach α 0.92 Support for new ideas (8 items) Cronbach α 0.90 Team Objective (11 items) Cronbach α 0.91 Task Orientation (7 items) Cronbach α 0.91 Reviewing Processes (7 items) Cronbach α 0.84 Social Relationships (8 items) Cronbach α 0.26	Watts, Lindqvist, Pearce, Drachler, and Richardson (2007)Anderson and West (1998)
Readiness for Interprofessional Learning Scale (RIPLS)	Focus on willingness for learners to learn together interprofessionally.	Professional identity Team-working	
Interdisciplinary Education Perception Scale (IEPS)	Focus on learners' level of comfort in learning together.	Competency and Autonomy. Internal consistency = 0.823 Perceived needs for professional cooperation. Internal consistency 0.56 Perception of actual cooperation. Internal consistency 0.54 Scale reliability Cronbach α 0.87	Developed by Luecht et al. (1990) Refined by McFadyen, Maclaren, and Webster (2007)

NAME OF INSTRUMENT	FOCUS OF MEASUREMENT	CONCEPTS ASSESSED	SOURCE
Interprofessional Praxis Audit Framework (IPAF)	Focus on organization's enactment of interprofessional practice.	Concepts: Context, culture, organization constructs (conduct – behavior, integration and interaction; attitudes – beliefs, values and philosophies; information – identification, representation, and distribution) Qualitative use of action research approach	Greenfield, Nugus, Travaglia, and Braithwaite (2010)
Assessment of Interprofessional Team Collaboration Scale (AITCS)	Focus on how team members see their team collaborating with each other and with clients and families.	Partnership/shared decision making (19 items) Cooperation (11 items) Coordination (7 items) Cronbach α 0.98	Orchard, King, Khalili, and Bezzina (2012)

Hence, team assessments must be made in concert with the realities of support for their interprofessional client-centered collaborative practice. A team that is still effective despite limited organizational support is more likely to experience more frustrations with their teamwork, especially when trying to work across units. Hence, such assessments, when made, can also be used to assist managers to advocate for changes in teamwork support at the organizational level.

Measurement of Team Interprofessional Client-Centered Collaborative Practice

Organizations that have made a commitment to interprofessional client-centered collaborative practice across all service areas may choose to track changes in client care outcomes from pre- to post-change to gain a comprehensive perspective of teamwork effectiveness.

An ideal way to enact such an assessment is through the use of instruments that have undergone rigorous psychometric analyses for both their validity and reliability. A number of instruments are available for such use and are listed below.

The information provided above is not an exhaustive listing of instruments to measure collaboration in teams, but a set of instruments that have been used with practitioners in practice settings that might be of value to organizations seeking to gain an evaluation of institution-wide teamwork. It is recommended that the developers of these instruments be contacted prior to considering their use to ensure the measure will fit with the goal for this assessment.

CONCLUSION

In this chapter a variety of strategies and concepts have been shared that may be used to assist the CIPE facilitator in assessing performance of practitioners and teams to enhance their collaborative teamwork as an outcome of CIPE program learning. The discussion provided a cycle from learning achieved through a CIPE program, to the conversion of this learning into transferable knowledge to a team, followed by the choice of uptake of this new knowledge into practice or not.

A number of selected approaches and concepts to assess were provided for assessment of performance at both the individual team member and team level. A discussion of the use of both process (formative) and outcomes (summative) approaches to assessment was provided and how these may be combined. A case was also made for assessing not only a team and its effectiveness, but also the support provided by organizations for collaborative teamwork. Finally, a number of instruments were shared that may be used to provide an overall assessment of collaborative teamwork across an organization.

REFERENCES

Anderson, N.R., and West, M.A. (1998). Measuring climate for work group innovation: development and validation of the team climate inventory. *Journal of Organizational Behavior, 19*, 235-258.

Attitudes toward Health Care Teams Scale. *Evaluation of Health Professionals, 22(1), 123-142.*

Bleakley, A. (2006). Broadening conceptions of learning in medical education: The message from teamworking. *Medical Education, 40,* 150–157. http://dx.doi.org/10.1111/j.1365-2929.2005.02371.x.

Boud, D. (2000). Sustainable assessment: Rethinking assessment for the learning society. *Studies in Continuing Education, 22,* 151–167. http://dx.doi.org/10.1080/713695728.

Canadian Interprofessional Health Collaborative. (2010). *A national interprofessional competency framework.* Retrieved from http://www.cihc.ca/files/CIHC_IPCompetencies_Feb1210.pdf.

Cohen, S.G., and Bailey, D.E. (1997). What makes teams work: Group effectiveness research from the shop floor to the executive suite. *Journal of Management, 23*(3), 239-290. doi: 10.1177/014920639702300303.

D'Amour, D., Goulet, L., Labadie, J.-F., San Martín-Rodríguez, L., and Pineault, R. (2008). A model and typology of collaboration between professionals in healthcare organizations. *BMC Health Services Research, 8,* 188–202. http://dx.doi.org/10.1186/1472-6963-8-188.

Dowding, D., and Thompson, C. (2003). Measuring the quality of judgment and decision-making in nursing. *Journal of Advanced Nursing, 44,* 49–57. http://dx.doi.org/10.1046/j.1365-2648.2003.02770.x.

Field, R., and West, M. A. (1995). Teamwork in primary health care. 2. Perspectives form practices. *Journal of Interprofessional Care, 9,* 123–130. http://dx.doi.org/10.3109/13561829509047846.

Gittell, J. H., Godfrey, M., and Thistlethwaite, J. (2013). Interprofessional collaborative practice and relational coordination: Improving healthcare through relationships. *Journal of Interprofessional Care, 27,* 210–213. http://dx.doi.org/10.3109/13561820.2012.730564.

Greenfield, D., Nugus, P., Travaglia, J., and Braithwaite, J. (2010). Auditing an organization's interprofessional learning and interprofessional practice: The interprofessional praxis audit framework (IPAF). *Journal of Interprofessional Care, 24,* 436–449. http://dx.doi.org/10.3109/13561820903163801

Heinemann, G.D., Schmidtt,M.H., Farrell, M.P., and Brallier, S.A. (1999). Development of an Interprofessional Education Collaborative. (2011). *Core competencies for interprofessional collaborative practice.* Retrieved from https://www.umassmed.edu/Global/Office%20of%20Educational%20Affairs/IPEG/CollaborativePractice.pdf.pdf.

Janhonen, M., and Johanson, J.-E. (2011). Role of knowledge conversion and social networks in team performance. *International Journal of Information Management 31,* 217–225. http://dx.doi.org/10.1016/j.ijinfomgt.2010.06.007.

Jeffery, A. B., Maes, J. D., and Bratton-Jeffery, M. F. (2005). Improving team decision-making performance with collaborative modeling. *Team Performance Management: An International Journal, 11*(1/2), 40–50. http://dx.doi.org/10.1108/13527590510584311.

King, G., Shaw, L., and Orchard, C. A., and Miller, S. (2010). The interprofessional socialization and valuing scale: A tool for evaluating the shift toward collaborative care approaches in health care settings. *Work: Journal of Prevention, Assessment and Rehabilitation, 35*, 77–85. http://dx.doi.org/10.3233/WOR-2010-0959.

Kvarnström, S. (2008). Difficulties in collaboration: A critical incident study of interprofessional healthcare teamwork. *Journal of Interprofessional Care, 22*, 191–203. http://dx.doi.org/10.1080/13561820701760600.

Lamb, B. W., Wong, H. W. L., Vincent, C., Green, J. S. A., and Sevdalis, N. (2011). Teamwork and team performance in multidisciplinary cancer teams: Development and evaluation of an observational assessment tool. *BMJ Quality and Safety, 20*, 849–856. http://dx.doi.org/10.1136/bmjqs.2010.048660.

Lavé, J. (2009). The practice of learning. In K. Illeris (Ed.), *Contemporary theories of learning: Leaning theorists in their own words* (pp. 200–208). London, United Kingdom: Routledge.

Légaré, F., Stacey, D., Pouliot, S., Gauvin, F.-P., Desroches, S., Kryworuchko, J., Graham, I. D. (2011). Interprofessionalism and shared decision-making in primary care: A stepwise approach towards a new model. *Journal of Interprofessional Care, 25*, 18–25. http://dx.doi.org/10.3109/13561820.2010.490502.

Lencioni, P. (2002). *The five dysfunctions of a team: A leadership fable.* San Francisco, CA: Jossey-Bass.

Lindqvist, S., Duncan, A., Shepstone, L., Watts, F., and Pearce, S. (2005). Development of the 'attitudes to health professionals questionnaire' (AHPQ): A measure to assess interprofessional attitudes. *Journal of Interprofessional Care, 19*(3), 269–279. http://dx.doi.org/10.1080/13561820400026071.

Luecht R, Madsen M, Taugher M, Petterson B. (1990). Assessing professional perceptions: design and validation of an interdisciplinary education perception scale. *J Allied Health. Spring*: 181–91.

Mathieu, J. E., Heffner, T. S., Goodwin, G. F., Salas, E., and Cannon-Bowers, J. A. (2000). The influence of shared mental models on team process and performance. *Journal of Applied Psychology, 85*, 273–283. http://dx.doi.org/10.1037/0021-9010.85.2.273.

McFadyen, A. K., Maclaren, W. M., and Webster, V. S. (2007). The interdisciplinary education perception scale (IEPS): An alternative remodelled sub-scale structure and its reliability. *Journal of Interprofessional Care, 21*, 433–443. http://dx.doi.org/10.1080/13561820701352531.

Orchard, C. A., Anderson, E., Ford, J. and Moran, M. (2015). *Framework for the Interprofessional Collaboration Judgment Assessment Tool.* Unpublished work.

Orchard, C. A., King, G. A., Khalili, H., and Bezzina, M. B. (2012). Assessment of Interprofessional Collaborative Practice (AITCS): Development and testing of the instrument. *Journal of Continuing Education in the Health Professions, 32*, 58–67. http://dx.doi.org/10.1002/chp.21123.

Pearson, D., and Pandya, H. (2006). Shared learning in primary care: Participants' views of the benefits of this approach. *Journal of Interprofessional Care, 20*, 302–313. http://dx.doi.org/10.1080/13561820600649672.

Pollard, K. C. (2008). Non-formal learning and interprofessional collaboration in health and social care: The influence of the quality of staff interaction on student learning about collaborative behavior in practice placements. *Learning in Health and Social Care, 7,* 12–26. http://dx.doi.org/10.1111/j.1473-6861.2008.00169.x.

Robinson, F. P., Gorman, G., Slimmer, L. W., and Yudkowsky, R. (2010). Perceptions of effective and ineffective nurse-physician communication in hospitals. *Nursing Forum, 45,* 206–216. http://dx.doi.org/10.1111/j.1744-6198.2010.00182.x.

Salas, E., Cooke, N. J., and Rosen, M. A. (2008). On teams, teamwork, and team performance: Discoveries and developments. *Human Factors, 50,* 540–547. http://dx.doi.org/10.1518/001872008X288457.

Salas, E., Rosen, M. A., Burke, C. S., Nicholson, D., and Howse, W. R. (2007). Markers for enhancing team cognition in complex environments: The power of team performance diagnosis. *Aviation, Space, and Environmental Medicine, 78*(Suppl. 5), B77–B85.

San Martín-Rodríguez, L., Beaulieu, M.-D., D'Amour, D., and Ferrada-Videla, M. (2005). The determinants of successful collaboration: A review of theoretical and empirical studies. *Journal of Interprofessional Care, 19*(Suppl. 1), 132–147. http://dx.doi.org/10.1080/13561820500082677.

Schön, D. A. (1991). *The reflective practitioner: How professionals think in action.* Aldershot, United Kingdom: Ashgate.

Watts, F., Lindqvist, S., Pearce, S., Drachler, M., and Richardson, B. (2007). Introducing a post-registration interprofessional learning programme for healthcare teams. *Medical Teacher, 29,* 443–449. http://dx.doi.org/10.1080/01421590701513706.

AUTHOR INDEX

A

Alford, J. (2009).

Allport, G. W. (1954).

Abma, T. A., & Broerse, J. E. W. (2009). (chapter 1)

Abu-Rish, E., Kim, S., Choe, L., Varpio, L., Malik, E., White, A. A., & Zierler, B. (2012). (chapter 8)

Adams, J. M., Hanesiak, R., Morgan, G., Owston, R., Lupshenyuk, D., & Mills, L. (2009). (chapter 8)

Adams, J. M., & Morgan, G. (2007). (chapter 8)

Adams, T. L., Orchard, C., Houghton, P., & Ogrin, R. (2014). (chapter 2)

Adler, R. B., & Proctor, R. F., II. (2010). (chapter 2)

Alford, J. (2009) (chapter 12)

American Association of the Colleges of Nursing and the Association of American Medical Schools (chapter 8)

B

Baker, G. R., Norton, P. G., Flintoft, V., Blais, R., Brown, A., Cox, J., . . . Tamblyn, R. (2004). (chapter 2, 7)

Bainbridge, L., Naismith, L., Orchard, C., & Wood, V. I. (2010). (chapter 3, 7)

Bainbridge, L., & Wood, V. I. (2013). (chapter 8)

Baldwin, A. (2013) (chapter 10)

Baldwin, D. C., & Daugherty, S. R. (2008). (chapter 7)

Balmer, J. T. (2012). (chapter 8)

Balmer, J. T. (2013). (chapter 8)

Bandura, A. (1988). (chapter 10)

Barello, S., Graffigna, G., & Vegni, E. (2012). (Introduction, chapter 1)

Barr, H. (2010). (chapter 6)

Barr, H. (2005) (chapter 5)

Barr, H., Koppel, I., Reeves, S., Hammick, M., & Freeth, D. (2005). (chapter 6, 10)

Bass, B. (1985). (chapter 3, 9)

Beach, M. C., & Inui, T. (2006). (chapter 1)

Bechtel, C., & Ness, D. L. (2010). (chapter 9)

BEME Collaboration (2012) (chapter 10)

Bernstein, B. (1971) (chapter 10)

Best Evidence Medical Education Collaboration. (2012). (chapter 10)

Billett, S. R. (2014) (chapter 8)

Bleakley, A. (2006). (chapter 3, 12)

Bono, J. E., & Judge, T. A. (2004). (Chapter 9)

Boud, D. (2015). (chapter 6, 12)

Bourdieu, P. (1997). (chapter 10)

Brandt, B. F., Quake-Rapp, C., Shanedling, J., Spannaus-Martin, D., & Martin, P. (2010). (chapter 8)

Brewer, M. L., & Jones, S. (2013) (chapter 5)

Briggs Myers, I., & Myers, P. B. (1995). (chapter 10)

Bushe, G. R., & Kassam, A. F. (2005) (chapter 5)

Chesluk, B. J., Reddy, S., Hess, B., Bernabeo, E., Lynn, L., & Holmboe, E. (2015)

C

CAIPE. (2002). (chapter 7)

Campbell, J. C., Coben, J. H., McLoughlin, E., Dearwater, S., Nah, G., Glass, N., et al. (2001). (chapter 6)

Canadian Health Services Research Foundation. (2006). (chapter 7)

Canadian Institute for Health Research. (2014). (chapter 8, 10)

Canadian Interprofessional Health Collaborative. (2008). (chapter 2, 8)

Canadian Interprofessional Health Collaborative. (2010). (introduction, chapter 2, 5, 7, 8, 10, 12)

Carlile, P. R. (2004). (chapter 10, 12)

Carman, K. L., Dardess, P., Maurer, M., Sofaer, S., Adams, K., Bechtel, C., & Sweeney, J. (2013). (chapter 1)

Carney, B. T., West, P., Neily, J., Mills, P. D., & Bagian, J. P. (2010) (chapter 3).

Carpenter, J., & Barnes, D. (2010) (chapter 3)

Dickson, C., & Wooff, D. (2006). (chapter 11)

Carpenter, J., Schneider, J., Brandon, T., & Wooff, D. (2003). (Introduction)

Carson, J. B., Tesluk, P. E., & Marrone, J. A. (2007). (chapter 2)

CASP (2012) (chapter 10)

Centre for the Advancement of Interprofessional Education (2002) (chapter 6, 8)

Center for Theory of Change. (2013). (chapter 11)

Charles, G., Bainbridge, L., & Gilbert, J. (2010). (chapter 8, 9)

Cheater, F. M., Hearnshaw, H., Baker, R., & Keane, M. (2005).

Cheetham, G., & Chivers, G. (1996). (chapter 2)

Chesluk, B. J., Reddy, S., Hess, B., Bernabeo, E., Lynn, L., & Holmboe, E. (2015). (chapter 6)

Chevalier, R. (2014). (chapter 8)

Chou, S. (2009) (chapter 5)

Cilliers, P. (1998). (chapter 10)

Clancy, C. M. (2011). (chapter 1)

Clark, P. G. (2009). (chapter 5, 10)

Clifton, M., Dale, C., & Bradshaw, C. (2007). (chapter 10)

Coffey, S., & Anyonam, C. (2015). (chapter 5)

Coffman, J. (1999). (chapter 11)

Coe, R., & Gould, D. (2008). (chapter 3)

Cohen, S. G., & Bailey, D. E. (1997). (Introduction, chapter 12)

Conn, L. G., Lingard, L., Reeves, S., Miller, K. L., Russell, A., & Zwarenstein, M. (2009). (chapter 2)

Cooperrider, D. L., & Whitney, D. (2005). (chapter 5, 11)

Correll, S. J. and Ridgeway, C. L. (2006). (chapter 10)

Costa, A. C. (2003). (chapter 2)

Coulter, A. (1999). (chapter 1)

Coulter, A. (2012). (chapter 1)

Coulter, A., & Ellins, J. (2007). (Introduction, chapter 3)

Craddock, D., Halloran, C. O., Mcpherson, K., Hean, S., Hammick, M., & O'Halloran, C. (2013). (chapter 10)

Cranston, P. (2011). (chapter 5)

Critical Appraisal Skills Programme. (2012). (chapter 10)

Curran, V., Deacon, D. R., & Fleet, L. (2005). (chapter 9)

Curran, V., Sargeant, J., & Hollett, A. (2007). (chapter 8)

Curran, V. (2006).

D

D'Amour, D., Goulet, L., Labadie, J.-F., San Martín-Rodríguez, L., & Pineault, R. (2008). (chapter 7)

D'Amour, D., & Oandasan I. (2005). (chapter 5,8)

David, G., Gunnarsson, C. L., Waters, H. C., Horblyuk, R., & Kaplan, H. S. (2013).

Davis, C. (2009). (chapter 3)

Davis, D. A., Mazmanian, P., Fordis, M., Harrison, R. V., Thorpe, K., & Perrier, L. (2006). (chapter 6)

Deneckere, S., Robyns, N., Vanhaecht, K., Euwema, M., Panella, M., Lodewijckx, C., . . . Sermeus, W. (2011). (Introduction, chapter 2, 7)

D'Eon, M. (2005). (chapter 5, 8)

Derouen, C., & Kleiner, B. H. (1994). (chapter 2)

Dowding, D., & Thompson, C. (2003). (chapter 12)

Drinka, T. J. K., & Clark, P. G. (2000). (Preface)

Dudek, J. G. (2012). (chapter 8)

Dzakiria, H., Wahab, M. S. D. A., & Rahman, H. D. A. (2012). (chapter 8)

E

Engeström, Y. (2001). (chapter 10)

Epstein, R. M., & Hundert, E. M. (2002). (chapter 2)

Eraut, M. (2003). (chapter 10)

Eraut, M. (2004). (chapter 8)

Erdem, F., & Ozen, J. (2003). (chapter 2)

Etchells, E., Mittmann, N., Koo, M., Baker, M., Krahn, M., Shojania, K., . . . Daneman, N. (2012). (chapter 7)

Eva, K., & Regehr, G. (2005). (chapter 6)

Eva, K., Regehr, G., & Gruppen, L. (2012). (chapter 6)

Excellent Care for All Act, 2010, RSO, 2010, c 14 [Ontario, Canada]. (Introduction)

Ezell, M. (2002). (chapter 5)

F

Fay, D., Borrill, C., Amir, S., Haward, R., & West, M. A. (2006). (Introduction)

Fawcett, J. (2005). (chapter 10)

Fawcett, J. (2003). (chapter 10)

Fawcett, J., & Downs, F. S. (1992) (chapter 10)

Festinger, L. (1957). (chapter 2, 10,

Field, R., & West, M. A. (1995). (chapter 12)

Fisher, W. R. (1987). (chapter 10)

Fitzpatrick, J. L., Sanders, J. R., & Worthen, B. R. (2004) (chapter 11)

Fleissig, A., Jenkins, V., Catt, S., & Fallowfield, L. (2006). (Introduction)

Florin, J., Ehrenberg, A., & Ehnfors, M. (2008). (chapter 1)

Flottorp, S. A., Oxman, A. D., Krause, J., Musila, N. R., Wensing, M., Godycki-Cwirko, M., Baker, R., & Eccles, M. P. (2013). (chapter 8)

Forsetlund, L. Bjørndal, A., Rashidian, A., Jamtvedt, G., O'Brien, M. A., Wolf, F. M., et al. (2009). (chapter 6)

Francis, R. (2013). (Chapter 6)

Frank, C., Asp, M., & Dahlberg, K. (2008). (chapter 1)

Frank, J. R., Snell, L. S., & Sherbino, J. (Eds.). (2015, March). (chapter 2)

Frank, J. R., Snell, L. S., Ten Cate, O., Holmboe, E. S., Carraccio, C., Swing, S. R., . . . Harris, K. A. (2010). (chapter 2)

Fraser, S. W., & Greenhalgh, T. (2001). (Introduction, chapter 2, 8, 10)

Freeth, D., Hammick, M., Koppel, I., Reeves, S., & Barr, H. (2002) (chapter 10)

Freeth, D., & Reeves, S. (2004). (chapter 11)

Freidson, E. (1970). (chapter 10)

Frenk, J., Bhutta, Z. A., Chen, L., Cohen, J., Crisp, N., Evans, T., Fineberg, H., . . . Zurayk, H. (2010). (chapter 8)

Fireire, P. (2002). (chapter 5)

Fudge, N., Wolfe, C. D. A., & McKevitt, C. (2008). (Introduction)

G

Gaboury, I. M., Lapierre, L., Boon, H., & Moher, D. (2011). (chapter 7)

Garrison, D. R. (2007). (chapter 8)

Garrison, R., Cleveland-Innes, M., & Vaughan, M. (n.d.). (chapter 8)

Garavan, T. N., & McGuire, D. (2001). (Introduction, chapter 2)

Garling P. (2008). (chapter 6)

Gilbert, J. (2005). (chapter 3, 9)

Gillespie, B. M., & Hamlin, L. (2009). (chapter 3)

Gittell, J. H., Godfrey, M., & Thistlethwaite, J. (2013). (Introduction, Chapter 1, 2, 12)

Goffman. (1963). (chapter 10)

Goh, S. C., Chan, C., & Kuziemsky, C. (2013). (chapter 7)

Goldman, J., Meuser, J., Rogers, J., Lawrie, L., & Reeves, S. (2010). (chapter 7)

Graham, I. D, Logan, J., Harrison, M. B., Straus, S.E., Tetore, J., Caswell. W., et al. (2006). (chapter 6)

Grant, C., Bainbridge, L., & Gilbert, J. (2010). (chapter 9)

Greenfield, D., Nugus, P., Travaglia, J., and Braithwaite, J. (2010). (chapter 11, 12)

Greenhalgh, T., & Macfarlane, F. (1997). (chapter 2)

Griscti, O., & Jacono, J. (2006). (chapter 6)

Gruman, J., Rovner, M. H., French, M. E., Jeffress, D., Sofaer, S., Shaller, D., & Prager, D. J. (2010). (Introduction, chapter 1)

H

Hall, P. (2005). (chapter 7, 9)

Hammick, M. (1998). (chapter 10)

Health Improvement and Innovation Resource Centre (2014). (chapter 3)

Health Professions Regulatory Advisory Council (2009). (chapter 5)

Headrick, L. A., Wilcock, P. M., & Batalden, P. B. (1998). (chapter 8)

Hean, S. (2014) (chapter 10)

Hean, S., Anderson, E., Bainbridge, L., Clark, P. G., Craddock, D., Doucet, S., Hammick, M., Mpofu, R., O'Halloran, C., Pitt, R., Oandasan, I. (2013) (chapter 10)

Hean, S., Craddock, D., & Hammick, M. (2012) (chapter 10)

Hean, S., Craddock, D., & O'Halloran, C. (2009). (chapter 10)

Hean, S., & Dickinson, C. S. (2005). (chapter 10)

Hean, S., Hammick, M., Miers, M., Barr, H., Hind, M., Craddock, D., Borthwick, A. and O'Halloran, C. (2009) (chapter 10)

Hean, S., O'Halloran, C., Craddock, D., Pitt, R., Anderson, L., & Morris, D. (2012). (chapter 10)

Hean, S., O'Halloran, C., Craddock, D., Hammick, M., & Pitt, R. (2013). (chapter 8)

Hean, S., et al (in review) (chapter 10)

Healey, A. N., Undre, S., & Vincent, C. A. (2006). (chapter 3)

Heinemann, G.D., Schmidt,M.H., Farrell, M.P., and Brallier, S.A. (1999). (chapter 12)

Helme, M., Jones, I., & Colyer, H. (2005) (chapter 10)

Henderson, S. (2003). (chapter 1)

Herbert, C. (2005). (chapter 5)

Hewstone, M. Brown, R. J. (1986). (chapter 10)

Headrick, L. A., Wilcock, P. M., & Batalden, P. B. (1998). (chapter 7)

Hibbard, J. H., Mahoney, E. R., Stock, R., & Tusler, M. (2007). (chapter 1, 2)

Ho, K., Jarvis-Selinger, S., Norman, C. D., Li, L. C., Olatunbosun, T., Cressman, C., & Nguyen, A. (2010). (chapter 8)

Hoffman, S. J., & Frenk, J. (2012). (chapter 8)

Hoffman, S. J., Rosenfield, D., Gilbert, J. H. V., & Oandasan, I. F. (2008). (chapter 9)

Howe, A., Billingham, K., & Walters, C. (2002). (chapter 8)

Howarth, M., Warner, H., & Haigh, C. (2012) (chapter 2)

Hughes, C. M., & McCann, S. (2003). (chapter 9)

I

IBM Corp. (2014a). (chapter 7)

IBM Corp. (2014b). (chapter 7)

Illeris, K. (2009). (chapter 10)

Interprofessional Education Collaborative. (2011). (chapter 12)

Interprofessional Education Collaborative Expert Panel. (2011). (chapter 10)

Institute of Medicine. (2001). (chapter 2)

Institute of Medicine. (2010). (chapter 8)

Institute of Medicine. (2015). (chapter 10)

Intercessional All Care Advisory Group (2006). (chapter 5)

Interprofessional Care Strategic Implementation Committee (2010). (chapter 5)

Interprofessional Education Collaborative Expert Panel (2011) (chapter 5)

IN-2-THEORY. [ca. 2010]. (chapter 10)

J

Janhonen, M., & Johanson, J.-E. (2011). (chapter 12)

Jary, D. J., & Jary, J. (1995). (chapter 10)

Jarvis, P. (2012). (chapter 1)

Jefffery, A. B., Maes, J. D., & Bratton-Jeffery, M. F. (2005). (chapter 12)

Johnson, H. L., & Kimsey, D. (2012). (chapter 3)

Jones (2000). (chapter 3)

K

Kanter, K. M. (1977). (chapter 7)

Kanter, K. M. (1993). (chapter 7)

Kaplan, S. (n.d.). (chapter 8)

Khomeiran, R. T., Yekta, Z. P., Kiger, A. M., & Ahmadi, F. (2006). (chapter 2)

Kim, J., Lowe, M., Srinivasan, V., Gairy, P., & Sinclair, L. (2010). (chapter 8)

Kim, K.-J., Bonk, C. J., & Oh, E. (2008). (chapter 8)

Kim, K.-J., Teng, Y.-T., Oh, E., & Cheng, J. (2008). (chapter 8)

King, G., Shaw, L, & Orchard, C. A., & Miller, S. (2010). (chapter 11, 12)

Kislov, R., Harvey, G., & Walshe, K. (2011). (chapter 8)

Kitto, S. C., Chesters, J., Thistlethwaite, J., & Reeves, S. (2011) (chapter 10)

Kitto, S. C., Bell, M., Goldman, J., Peller, J., Silver, I., Sargeant, J., & Reeves, S. (2013). (chapter 8)

Kohn, L. T., Corrigan, J. M., & Donaldson, M. S. (Eds.). (1999). (chapter 7)

Kolb, D. A. (1984). (chapter 10)

Kouzes, J. M., & Posner, B. Z. (2012). (chapter 2)

KT Clearinghouse. (n.d.). (chapter 8)

Kvarnström, S. (2008). (chapter 12)

L

Lamb, B. W., Wong, H. W. L., Vincent, C., Green, J. S. A., & Sevdalis, N. (2011). (chapter 12)

Lamb, B., & Clutton, N. (2012) (chapter 3)

Laschinger, H. K. S., Read, E., Wilk, P., & Finegan, J. (2014). (chapter 7)

Laschinger, H. K. S., & Smith, L. M. (2013). (chapter 7)

Lavé, J. (2009). (chapter 12)

Lavé, J., & Wenger, E. (1991). (chapter 6)

Lawrence, R. L. (2002). (chapter 8)

LeCornu, A. (2009). (chapter 1)

Le Deist, F. D., & Winterton, J. (2005). (chapter 2)

Lee, H.-J. (2004). (chapter 2)

Lee, J. (2010). (chapter 8)

Lee, S.-Y. D., Arozullah, A. M., & Cho, Y. K. (2004). (chapter 1)

Leeman, J., Baernholdt, M., & Sandelowski, M. (2007). (chapter 8)

Légaré, F., Borduas, F., Macleod, T. Sketris, I., Campbell, B., & Jacques, A. (2011). (chapter 8)

Légaré, F., Freitas, A., Thompson-Deduc, P., Borduas, F., Luconi, F., Boucher, A. et al. (2014). (chapter 6)

Légaré, F., Stacey, D., Pouliot, S., Gauvin, F.-P., Desroches, S., Kryworuchko, J., Dunn, S., Elwyn, G., Frosch, D., Gagnon, M.-P., Harrison, M. B., Pluye, P., & Graham, I. D. (2011). (chapter 12)

Lencioni, P. (2002). (chapter 12)

Lequerica, A. H., Donnell, C. S., & Tate, D. G. (2009). (Introduction)

Lees, A., & Meyer, E. (2011). (chapter 8)

Li, L. C., Grimshaw, J. M., Nielsen, C., Judd, M., Coyte, P. C., & Graham, I. D. (2009). (chapter 8)

Lingard, L., Espin, S., Whyte, S., Regehr, G., Baker, G. R., Reznick, R., . . . Grober, E. (2004). (chapter 3)

Lingard, L., Garwood, S., & Poenaru, D. (2004). (chapter 3)

Lingard, L., Vanstone, M., Durrant, M., Fleming-Carroll, B., Lowe, M., Rashotte, J., . . . Tallett, S. (2012). (chapter 7)

Lindqvist, S., Duncan, A., Shepstone, L., Watts, F., & Pearce, S. (2005). (chpater 12)

Lown, B. A., & Manning, C. F. (2010). (chapter 7)

Lingard, L., Vanstone, M., Durrant, M., Fleming-Carroll, B., Lowe, M., Rashotte, J., . . . Tallett, S. (2012). (chapter 7)

Longtin, Y., Sax, H., Leape, L. L., Sheridan, S. E., Donaldson, L., & Pittet, D. (2010). (chapter 1)

Lotrecchiano, G. R., McDonald, P. L., Lyons, L., Long, T., & Zajicek-Farber, M. (2013). (chapter 8)

Lown, B. A., & Manning, C. F. (2010). (chapter 7)

Luecht R, Madsen M, Taugher M, Petterson B. (1990). (chapter 12)

M

Macdonald, M. B., Bally, J. M., Ferguson, L. M., Lee Murray, B., Fowler-Kerry, S. E., & Anonson, J. M. S. (2010). (chapter 2)

Mansfield, R. (2004). (chapter 2)

Manley, K., Titchen, A., Hardy, S. (2009). (chapter 8)

Mann, K., Gordon, J., & MacLeod, A. (2009). (chapter 5)

Mansour, M. (2009). (chapter 7)

Marshal, R. J., & Grant, D. (2008). (chapter 5)

Martin, G. P. (2011). (chapter 1)

Martin, G. P., & Finn, R. (2011).

Mazzocco, K., Petitti, D. B., Fong, K. T., Bonacum, D., Brookey, J., Graham, S., . . . Thomas, E. J. (2009). (chapter 7)

McNair, R. P. (2005). (Introduction, chapter 2)

Mathieu, J. E., Goodwin, G. F., Heffner, T. S., Salas, E., & Cannon-Bowers, J. A. (2000). (chapter 12)

McFadyen, A. K., MacLaren, W. M., & Webster, V. S. (2007). (chapter 12)

McCallin, A. (2003) (chapter 10)

Merriam, S. B., & Leahy, B. (2005). (chapter 8)

Meuser, J., Bean, T., Goldman, J., & Reeves, S. (2006). (chapter 5)

Mezirow, J. (1999). (chapter 5)

Mezirow, J. (1997). (chapter 10)

Mickan, S. M., & Rodger, S. A. (2005). (chapter 10)

Miller, B. M., Moore, D. E. Jr., Stead, W. W., & Balser, J. R. (2010). (chapter 8)

Mitchell, R., Parker, V., Giles, M., & Boyle, B. (2014). (chapter 7)

Moore, D. R., Cheng, M.-I., & Dainty, A. R. J. (2002). (chapter 2)

Moore, D. E., Green, J. S., & Gallis, H. A. (2009). (chapter 8)

Moore, D. E., Green, J. S., Jay, S. J., Leist, J. C., & Maitland, F. M. (1994). (chapter 8)

Morey, J. C., Simon, R., Jay, G. D., Wears, R. L., Salisbury, M., Dukes, K. A., et al. (2002). (chapter 6)

Morris, Z. S., Woodings, S., & Grant, J. (2011). (chapter 6)

Moss-Morris. R., Weinman. K., Petree, L. K., Horne, R., Cameron, L. D., & Buick. D. (2002). (chapter 1)

Myers (1980, 1995). (chapter 10)

N

National Health Service and Community Care Act, 1990, c. 19 [United Kingdom]. (Introduction)

Nelson, S., Tassone, M., & Hodges, B. D. (2014). (chapter 5)

Nembhard, I. M., & Edmondson, A. C. (2006). (chapter 7)

New Zealand Code of Health and Disability Services Consumer' Rights (1996). (chapter 3)

Nisbet, G., Lincoln, M., & Dunn, S. (2013). (chapter 8)

Northouse, P. G. (2001). (chapter 10)

Nugus, P., Greenfield, D., Travaglia, J., Westbrook, J., & Braithwaite, J. (2010). (Introduction)

O

Oandasan, I. (2006). (chapter 5)

Oandasan, I., & Barker, K. (2003). (chapter 5)

Oandasan, I., & Reeves, S. (2005). (chapter 5, 8)

Oandasan, I., Robinson, J., Bosco, C., Casimiro, L., Dorschner, D., & Schwartz, L. (2009). (chapter 5)

O'Brien, D., McCallin, A., & Bassett, S. (2013). (chapter 9)

Oelke, N., Cunning, L., Andrews, K., Martin, D., MacKay, A., Kuschminder, K., and Congdon, V. (2009). (chapter 8)

Orchard, C. A. (2008). (Introduction)

Orchard, C. A. (2009) (chapter 2)

Orchard, C. A. (2014). (chapter 2)

Orchard, C. A., Anderson, E., Ford, J., Moran, M. (2015). (chapter 12)

Orchard, C. A., Curran, V., & Kabene, S. (2005). (Introduction, chapter 2, 3, 8)

Orchard. C., King, G., Khalili, & Bezzina, M. B. (2012). (chapter 11, 12)

Orchard, C. A., & Rykhoff, M. (2015). (chapter 2)

Ottawa Hospital. (2007). (chapter 7)

P

Page, A. (2003). (chapter 7)

Parboosingh, I. J., Reed, V. A., Palmer, J. C., & Bernstein, H. H. (2011). (chapter 8)

Parker Oliver, D., Wittenberg-Lyles, E. M., & Day, M. (2007).

Parsons, T. (1951). (chapter 10)

Pawson, R., & Tilley, N. (1997). (chapter 10, 12)

Payler, J., Meyer, E., & Humphries, D. (2011). (chapter 8)

Pearce, C. L. (2004). (Introduction, chapter 2)

Pearce, C. L., & Sims, H. P., Jr. (2002). (chapter 2)

Pearson, D., & Pandya, H. (2006). (chapter 12)

Pettigrew, T. F. (1998). (Introduction)

Pettigrew, T. F., & Tropp, L. R. (2008). (Introduction)

Pearce, C. L., & Barkus, B. (2004). (chapter 2)

Pearce, C. L., & Sims, H. P., Jr. (2002). (chapter 2)

Pfaff, K., Baxter, P., Jack, S., & Ploeg, J. (2014). (chapter 7)

Pollard, K. C. (2008). (chapter 12)

Porter O'Grady, T. (2003). (chapter 10)

Poulton, B. C., & West, M. A. (1999). (chapter 7)

Prochaska, J. O., & Norcross, J. C. (2001). (chapter 1)

PROFRES. (2014) (chapter 10)

Pullon, S. (2008). (chapter 9)

R

Raab, C. A., Will, S. E. B., Richards, S. L., & O'Mara, E. (2013). (chapter 7)

Rabin, R. (2013). (chapter 8)

Ranmuthugala, G., Plumb, J. J., Cunningham, F. C., Georgiou, A., Westbrook, J. I., & Braithwaite, J. (2011). (chapter 8)

Reeves, S. (Ed.). (2013). (chapter 10)

Reeves, S., Perrier, L., Goldman, J., Freeth, D., & Zwarenstein, M. (2013). (chapter 6, 8)

Reeves, S., Macmillan, K., & van Soeren, M. (2010). (chapter 7)

Reeves, S., Zwarenstein, M., Goldman, J., Barr, H., Freeth, D., Hammick, M., et al. (2008). (chapter 6)

Reeves, S., Fox, A., & Hodges, B. D. (2009). (chapter 2)

Regan, S., Laschinger, H. K. S., & Wong, C. A. (2015). (chapter 7)

Registered Nursing Association of Ontario. (2006). (chapter 8)

Regulated Health Professions Act, 1991, RS 1991, c 18 [Ontario]. (chapter 5)

Ridgeway, C. L. (2001). (chapter 10)

Ridgeway, C. L. (2006). (chapter 10)

Ridgeway, C. L. (2011). (chapter 10)

Riegel, B., Jaarsma, T., & Strömberg, A. (2012). (Introduction, chapter 1, 2)

Rittel, H. W. J., & Webber, M. M. (1973). (Preface)

Robinson, F. P., Gorman, G., Slimmer, L. W., & Yudkowsky, R. (2010). (chapter 2, 12)

Roegiers, X. (2007). (Introduction, chapter 2)

Rosen, M. A., Hunt, E. A., Pronovost, P. J. Federowicz, M. A., & Weaver, S. J. (2012). (chapter 8,)

Rossett, A., & Frazee, R. V. (2006). (chapter 8)

Rydenfält, C., Johansson, G., Larsson, P. A., Åkerman, K., & Odenrick, P. (2012). (chapter 3)

S

Safran, D. G., Miller, W., & Beckman, H. (2006). (chapter 7)

Sahlsten, M. J. M., Larsson, I. E., Sjöström, B., & Plos, K. A. (2008). (chapter 1)

Sahlsten, M. J. M., Larsson, I. E., Sjöström, B., & Plos, K. A. (2009). (chapter 1)

Salas, E., DiazGrandos, D., Klien, C., Burke, S., Stagl, K. C., Goodwin, G. F., & Halpin, S. M. (2008). (chapter 7)

Salas, E., DiazGranados, D., Weaver, S. J., & King, H. (2008). (chapter 2, 12)

Salas, E., Rosen, M. A., Burke, C. S., Nicholson, D., & Howse, W. R. (2007). (chapter 12)

San Martín-Rodríguez, L. A., Beaulieu, M.-D., D'Amour, D., & Ferrada-Videla, M. (2005). (chapter 8, 12)

Sargeant, J. (2009). (chapter 8)

Sargeant, J., Borduas, F., Sales, A., Klein, D., Lynn, B., & Stenerson, H. (2011). (chapter 8)

Saunders, P. (1995). (chapter 1)

Scheming, E. H. (1993). (chapter 5)

Schön, D. A. (1991). (chapter 5, 12)

Sense, M. (2006). (chapter 5)

Sexton, M. E. (2014). (chapter 2)

Shields, P. (2003). (chapter 8)

Shortell, S. M., Rousseau, D. M., Gillies, R. R., Devers, K. J., & Simons, T. L. (1991). (chapter 7)

Shulman, A. S. (2005). (Introduction)

Simmons, B., & Wagner, S. (2009). (chapter 8)

Singh, H., & Reed, C. (2001). (chapter 8)

Solomon, P., Baptiste, S., Hall, P., Luke, R., Orchard, C., Rukholm, E., . . . Damiani-Taraba, G. (2010). (chapter 9)

Spouse, J. (2001). (chapter 8)

Stiles, K. A., Horton-Deutsch, S., & Andrews, C. A. (2014). (chapter 7)

Stoof, A., Martens, R. L., van Merriënboer, J. J. G., & Bastiaens, T. J. (2002). Suter, E., Arndt, J., Arthur, N., Parboosingh, J., Taylor, E., & Deutschlander, S. (2009). (chapter 2)

Stutsky, B. J., & Laschinger, H. K. S. (2014). (chapter 7)

Suter, E., Arndt, J., Arthur, N., Parboosingh, J., Taylor, E., & Deutschlander, S. (2009). (chapter 2, 10)

T

Tajfel, H. (1981). (chapter 10)

Tajfel, H., & Turner, J. C. (1986). (chapter 10)

Tardif, H. (1999). (chapter 2, 10)

Temkin-Greener, H., Gross, D., Kunitz, S. J., & Mukamel, D. (2004). (chapter 7)

Testing, D. T., & Jackson, S. F. (1994, April 5). (chapter 5)

Theory of Change. (n.d.). (chapter 11)

Turner, J. (1999). (chapter 10)

ten Cate, O., & Scheele, F. (2007). (chapter 2)

Thistlethwaite, J. (2012). (chapter 6)

Thistlethwaite, J., Jackson, A., & Moran, M. (2013). (Preface)

Thompson, R. S., Rivara, F. P., Thompson, D. C., Barlow, W. E., Sugg, N. K., Maiuro, R. D., et al. (2000). (chapter 6)

Tomson, R., Murtagh, M., & Khaw, F.-M. 2005). (chapter 1)

Travis, J. (2002). (chapter 2)

U

University of Western Ontario, Office of the Interprofessional Health Education & Research. (2014). (chapter 1, 2)

University of Western Ontario, Office of the Interprofessional Health Education & Research. (2015). (chapter 1, 2)

Urquhart, R., Cornelissen, E., Lal, S., Colquhoun, H., Klein, G., Richmond, S., & Witteman, H. O. (2013). (chapter 8)

V

Van Hoof, T. J., & Meehan, T. P. (2011). (chapter 8)

Vygotsky, L. (1978). (chapter 10)

W

Wackerhausen, S. (2009). (chapter 10)

Walker, D., & Nocon, H. (2007). (chapter 10)

Walsh, C. L., Gordon, M. F., Marshall, M., Wilson, F., & Hunt, T. (2005). (chapter 10)

Wang, M., Ran, W., Liao, J., & Yang, S. J. H. (2010). (chapter 8)

Watts, F., S. Lindqvist, S., Pearce, S., Drachler, M., & Richardson, B. (2007). (chapter 12)

Webster-Wright, A. (2009). (chapter 6)

Wenger-Trayner, E., & Wenger-Trayner, B. (2015). (chapter 8)

West, M. A., & Field, R. (1995). (chapter 2, 12)

Wilcock, P. M., Janes, G., & Chambers, A. (2009). (chapter 6)

Wilhelmsson, M., Pelling, S., Uhlin, L., Lars, O. D., Faresj, T., & Forslund, K. (2012) (chapter 10)

Woodall, D., & Hovis, S. (2013). (chapter 8)

World Health Organization. (1988). (chapter 6)

World Health Organization. (2006). (chapter 7)

World Health Organization. (2008). (chapter 3)

World Health Organization. (2010). (chapter 3, 5, 6, 7, 8, 10)

World Health Organization. (2012). (chapter 3)

World Health Organization. (2013). (chapter 8)

World Health Organization. (2014). (chapter 1)

Wyatt, Knowlton, L., & Phillips, C. C. (2013). (chapter 11)

Y

Yamnill, S., & Mclean, G. N. (2001). (chapter 8)

Young, A. S., Chinman, M., Forquer, S. L., Knight, E. L., Vogel, H., Miller, A., et al. (2005). (chapter 6)

Zwarenstein M., & Reeves S. (2006). (chapter 8)

Zweibel, E. B., Goldstein, R., Manwaring, J. A., & Marks, M. B. (2008). (chapter 2)

Z

Zwarenstein, M., Goldman, J., & Reeves, S. (2009). (chapter 7, 8)

SUBJECT INDEX

A

Abstracts 1, 14, 37, 51, 67, 83, 95, 114, 131, 143, 161, 171
Acknowledgements viii, 124
Accuracy 162
Addressing Differing Perceptions of Teamwork xx
Addressing Power Relationships between Health Provider Groups xxii
Advancing behavioral and leadership changes in practice settings 77
An Example of a Team Management Plan for Martha & Her Family 90
An Integrative Approach 25
Application of an Integrative Pedagogical Approach to Interprofessional Collaborative Practice 25
Approaches to Competency Frameworks 24
Assessment of Learning within Continuing Interprofessional Client-Centered Collaborative Practice 171
Assessment of Team Performance 178
Author Biographies x
Author index 189

B

Barriers to Interprofessional Learning and Practice 134
Background 132
Blended Learning 114
Building Social Capital 54

C

Case Study 11, 19, 39, 105, 132, 166
Case Study Analysis 12, 138

Case Study regarding Interprofessional Continuing Education Professional Development (CIPD) in the Workplace 120
Chapter 1. Towards a Framework of Client-Centered Collaborative Practice 1
Chapter 2. What is Competence in Client-Centered Collaborative Practice? Xxiv, 17
Chapter 3. Perioperative Practice in the Context of Client-Centered Care xxiv, 38
Chapter 4. Should there be an 'I' in Team? A New Perspective on Developing and Maintaining Collaborative Networks in Health Professional Care xxiv, 51
Chapter 5. Changing Organizational Culture to Embrace Interprofessional Education and Interprofessional Practice xxiv, 67
Chapter 6. Engaging Health Professionals in Continuing Interprofessional Development xxiv, 83
Chapter 7. The Effect of Leadership Support on Interprofessional Practice, Team Effectiveness, and Patient Safety Outcomes xxiv, 95
Chapter 8: Transformative Interprofessional Continuing Education and Professional Development to Meet Patient Care Needs: A Synthesis of Best Practices xxiv, 114
Chapter 9 Theory into Practice: The Challenges and Rewards of Developing and Running an Interprofessional Health Clinic xxiv, 131
Chapter 10. Moving from Atheoretical to Theoretical Approaches to Interprofessional Client-Centered Collaborative Practice xxiv, 143
Chapter 11. Evaluation of Continuing Interprofessional Client-Centered Collaborative Practice Programs xxiv, 161
Chapter 12. Assessment of Learning within Continuing Interprofessional Client-Centered Collaborative Practice xxiv, 171
CIPD to Promote Change 86
Client Activation 10

Client Engagement 3
Client Health Literacy 8
Client Health Provider Relationship 8
Client Participation 8
Clinical and Administrative Responsibilities 45
Changing the Organizational Culture to Embrace IPE
    and IPC 67
Client Engagement 3
Client Health Literacy 8
Client/Health Provider Relationships 8
Client Involvement in Their Care xxii
Client Participation 8
Clinical and Administrative Responsibilities 45
CIPD to Promote Change 86
Co-Creation Process 146
Co-Creation of Innovative Solutions to Practice
    Problems using Theory as a Tool 153
Collaborative & Shared Leadership 30
Communication 47
Communication means 180
Competency-based Frameworks 25
Complementary relationships 179
Conclusion 14, 32, 48, 61, 78, 91, 105, 124, 141,
    157, 169, 184
Consideration of Learning Context Is Important 115
    Context of Practice xviii
Creating a Learning Culture to Advance
    Interprofessional Client-Centered Care 70

D

Data Analysis 102
Descriptive Results 103
Designing Learning to Improve Knowledge 117
Determining When Learning Delivery Method(s) to
    Use Requires Careful consideration 116
Developing Consistent Levels of Skill Acquisition
    21
Discussion 59, 104, 169
Discussion and implications 41
Domain or Subject Competence 21

E

Education and government sectors advancement of
    structural changes 77
Education and Preparation 6
Embracing All Parts of the Whole in Advancing IPE
    and IPC 71
Empirical adequacy 155
Engaging Busy Professionals 87

Engaging Health Professionals in Continuing
    Interprofessional Development 83
Establishing Continuing Interprofessional Education
    46
Evaluation of Continuing Interprofessional Client-
    Centered Collaborative Practice Programs 161
Evidence for Effectiveness of Continuing
    Professional Development 84
Evidence for CIPD as Shared Learning 85
Evidence of Change 77

F

Feasibility 162
Findings 120
Foreword, vii

H

How Does the Patient or Client Fit into a Team? 6
How Clients Interacted with the Clinic 134

I

Identifying the content for CIPD 86
Impact of the Implemented Changes 136
Implications for Management 107
Implications for Practice 121
Individual 140
Institutional 138
Instruments 102
Interactional determinants 181
Interdependencies 179
Interprofessional Collaborative Practice in the
    Operating Theater 38
Interprofessional Collaboration 102
Interprofessional Communication 28
InterprofesionalCompetency Framework 179
Interprofessional Conflict Resolution 31
Interprofessional Education as a form of Advocacy
    68
IN-2-Theory as an International Community of
    Practice 145
Intra-Operative Phase 41
Intra-Operative Phase of the Interprofessional Client-
    Centered Experience 44
Introduction xvii, 1, 14, 37, 51, 67, 84, 96, 114, 131,
    143, 161, 171

K

Knowledge contribution of members 179

L

Leadership 97, 102
Learning as an Outcome of Continuing
    Interprofessional Education Training 174
Learning Assessment 172
Learning Delivery Methods 116
Life Skills-Based Frameworks 25
Limitations 105

M

Managing Conflict 58
Measurement of Impact 122
Measurement of the individual member of, or of the
    team? 174
Measurement of Team Interprofessional Client-
    Centered Collaborative Practice 184
Methods 53
Moving from Atheoretical to Theoretical
    Approaches to Interprofessional Client-Centered
    Collaborative Practice 143

N

Negotiating Priorities and Resources 57

O

Organizational boundaries 179
Organizational Environment 181
Organizational determinants 181
Overview of Book Chapters xxiii

P

Parsimony 154
Path Analysis Results 103
Patient/Client/Family/Community-based Care 27
Patient Safety 102
Pre-Operative Phase 39
PeriOperative Phase of the Interprofessional Client-
    Centered Care Experience 43
Perioperative Practice in the Context of Client-
    Centered Care 37

Personal Competence 23
Perspective Taking 56
Post-Operative Phase 43
Post-Operative Phase of the Interprofessional Client-
    Centered Care Experience 45
Practice Environment & Individual Fit 23
Practitioners Knowledge: The use of narrative 147
Pragmatic Adequacy 156
Preface
Pre-Operative Phase (chapter 3)
Pre-Operative Phase of the Interprofessional Client-
    Centered Care Experience 43
Procedures 100
Professional Socialization xxi
Program Evaluation 162
Program Logic Model Evaluation Approach 164
Propriety 162

R

References xxiv, 14, 33, 49, 62, 79, 92, 108, 124,
    141,157, 170, 185
Regulatory and government policy changes 78
Results 54, 103
Role Clarification 29

S

Should there be an 'I' in Team? A New Perspective
    on Developing and Maintaining Collaborative
    Networks in Health Professional Care 51
Skill-Based Competency Frameworks 24
Social Competence 23
Staff Capacity 137
Strategies to Address Client Case Issues in the
    Perioperative Setting 46
Student Interprofessional Learning Opportunities
    138
Subject Index 197
Summary of Workshop Model 156
Support Structures 102

T

Team 140
Team Dynamics 178
Team Effectiveness 102
Team Functioning 30
Team Practice Environment and Individual Fit 23
Teamwork 47
Testability 155

The Effect of Leadership Support on
   Interprofessional Practice, Team Effectiveness,
   and Patient Safety Outcomes 95
The Learning Context 115
The Patient or Client Connecting to a Collaborative
   Practice Model 7
The Story of Advancing Interprofessional Client-
   Centered Care in the Province of Ontario 72
The Workshop Model 146
Theoretical Framework 96
Theorists Knowledge 149
Theoretical Framework 100
Theoretical Adequacy 155
Theoretical Quality and Competence 154
Theory into Practice: The Challenges and Rewards
   of Developing and Running an Interprofessional
   Health Clinic 131
The Patient or Client Connecting to a Collaborative
   Practice Model 7
The Story of Advancing Interprofessional Client-
   Centered Care in the Province of Ontario 72
The Workshop Model 146

Towards a Framework of Client-Centered
   Collaborative Practice 1
Transfer Design 119
Transfer of Learning into Practice 176

U

Uni-disciplinary Education xxi
Use of a Case Study to Stimulate Discussion: The
   Case of Martha Schmidt 89
Using Educational Theories to Foster Change 69
Utility 161

W

What Can the Patient or Client do in a Team? 6
What is Competence in Client-Centered
   Collaborative Practice? 14
Who is a Patient or Client? 6
Workshop Aim 146
Workshop Participants 146